TAKING ON PARKINSON'S

BY

DENNIS JAY O'DONNELL

Copyright 2017 by Dennis Jay O'Donnell. All rights are reserved. A Domec, Inc. project.

No part of this book may be used or reproduced in any manner without written permission except in the case of brief quotations used in articles or reviews.

Cover design by For the Muse Designs
Edited/Formatted by Concierge Self-Publishing
(www.ConciergeSelfPublishing.com)

This book is dedicated to my wife, my love and life co-director, Mary Ellen Campbell,
whose mantra, "Do something outside your comfort zone every year,"
keeps me on point and ready for adventure.
With her at my side, never flinching in the face of change, the future is ours to make.

Table of Contents

Acknowledgements   i
Foreword   iii

INTRODUCTION

DIAGNOSIS

Chapter 1: The Parky Professor   17

UNCHARTED WATERS

Chapter 2: Finding a Neurologist Who Fits   25
Chapter 3: Medicine: Wild Thing   33
Chapter 4: Physical Therapy: A Creative Art   43
Chapter 5: The RGS4 Protein Needs Dopamine …   49

PREDICAMENTS

Chapter 6: "Oh, I Know Someone with Parkinson's"   61
Chapter 7: "We Don't Give Out Blankets Anymore."   67

EXERCISE

Chapter 8: Whiskey Friday   79

Chapter 9: I Always Wanted to Do That	83
Chapter 10: "Could You Dry This Off for Us?"	87
Chapter 11: "Okay, Everybody …	91

CHILDREN

Chapter 12: "Hey Mom …	103
Chapter 13: Little Man, Little Boy	107

INTERVENORS

Chapter 14: Hells Angels	115
Chapter 15: Intermission	121
Chapter 16: Fly Fishing in a Small World	127
Chapter 17: "I Can't Walk Just Now …	133
Chapter 18: "I'll Get You up the Stairs!"	139
Chapter 19: "I Used to Walk Like That …	143
Chapter 20: Do One Thing a Year that Is Scary	147
Chapter 21: These Are Not Real Tears	155
Chapter 22: Tap, Tap, Tap …	161
Chapter 23: I Don't Think Shaking It Will Fix It	165

GAINING PERSPECTIVE

Chapter 24: Looking Back	175
Chapter 25: Brain Surgery	191

DISCOVERING DBS SURGERY

Chapter 26: Doing the DBS   197

CONTINUING ON

Chapter 27: Survivor   205
Chapter 28: Looking Ahead   213

EPILOGUE

Acknowledgements

I would like to acknowledge the following people, family and friends who made a contribution to my efforts to write this book. None of its flaws are the responsibility of them; the errors remain mine alone.

My love to Daphne, Michael and my amazing grandchildren, Maddy, Allie, Nick and Rachel, who constantly take on the future with relish and great success. They simply inspire me.

To the Missoula handball group of gentlemen and tough as nails men, I raise a glass at Whiskey Friday to your enduring lesson that age is a condition of the mind. To Rod, Robo, Louie, Doc, Emmons, Wally, Tommy and scores of other worthy opponents, I know that the longer you play the better you were.

To the Wednesday men's reading group. As a matter of duty, you stayed intellectually alive to the search for knowledge at any age. Your wisdom is a collective good that helps me retain a sharp mind, just to keep up.

To my friends Marcy and Phil, Ian and Joanne, Paul and Beth, David and Sancia, Bente and Don, Don and Shirley, Harold and Jan and Ben Loehnen, Sharon and Dick, to name just a few who helped support my book efforts, thank you for being there.

To Robert Campbell and Tim O'Leary, my enduring gratitude for your commitment to me, Robert as my trusted nephew and young guardian and Tim as a fellow writer and dynamic example of how much can be really done if you put your mind and effort behind an idea. Each of you is invaluable to me.

To all those anonymous people whose acts of kindness are the grist for this book. It was my pleasure to see you in action when the situation called for your help. You appeared because the moment called you. I'm the lucky beneficiary of being in the right time and the right place when you acted on my behalf.

To all researchers and practitioners who have made Parkinson's disease (PD) your career. Without your efforts those with PD would have few alternatives to maintain meaningful lives. My thanks especially go out to Dr. Matt Brodsky and Dr. Sherry Reid, neurologists extraordinaire.

To Hadley Ferguson and Tom Seekins, people who are brave enough to face Parkinson's with great courage, and the Board of Directors of Summit for Parkinson's over the years. Keep up the good fight.

Foreword

"Taking on Parkinson's" is about my personal experience in dealing with Parkinson's disease (PD). Those of us who have Parkinson's, those who are working to assist us and partners of people with Parkinson's eventually come to the realization that it can't be controlled, negotiated with, prevented or cured at this time. When a person is first diagnosed with Parkinson's, the urge is to deny it or to be angry at it. After 16 years, I'm certain that the only thing that can be done is to attempt to take on Parkinson's for as long as possible.

Writing this book allowed me to sum up my experience about the human capacity to be creative and durable in the face of physical challenges. This act of recalling situations that challenged my patience and sometimes my capacities has given me confidence that Parkinson's and other movement disorders can often be corralled if not outmaneuvered. As I have observed others coping with PD and other movement disorders, I have often thought back to incidents when I gained an insight that helped me transcend the frustrations I felt at that moment.

SECTION 1: INTRODUCTION

Dealing with PD reminds me of a time when my father found me embroiled in a major fistfight with a willow bush that had grabbed my fishing line for the fourth time. I was 12, with the adrenaline and determination to conquer the world, but without the skills even to control myself.

I was dry fly fishing on a beautiful stream at the foot of the Collegiate Peaks in central Colorado. It should have been a serene and life affirming afternoon. Instead, I was fighting a huge willow bush as though I had come upon evil incarnate. Of course, I was losing. Thrashing was just making things worse.

Laughter rose above the sounds of breaking tree limbs. I was instantly furious at my father.

"I used to do that until I looked up and down the stream at the willows and realized I was severely outnumbered," he said. He spread his arms, looked up and down the stream and asked, "Butch, are you outnumbered?"

For a split second I glanced up and then down the stream, then sheepishly smiled. He grabbed and hugged me and ruffed up my hair as we both laughed. I learned a very important lesson that day.

People can't win against inanimate objects or stop an inexorable process. Rather, they are better served to laugh at the situation and learn something about dealing with the problem. From that day forward, whenever I had trouble I always heard my father's voice say, "Are you outnumbered?" and I'd know what to do: Take a moment to laugh and work around the problem instead of doing battle with it. Persevere. This important lesson about recognizing when we are outnumbered is my father's lasting reminder that it is my ability to decide to control my attitude toward a problem that gives me a chance to corral it.

That is how I have dealt with such a powerful force as Parkinson's.

Persevering in the Face of Parkinson's

Unfortunately, controlling one's attitude and naming the unknown is not enough to corral PD alone. Dealing with PD has required me to call on many people. Surprisingly, numerous volunteers have often shown up just when needed.

People rise to the occasion when they see someone engaged in a battle with body control. Almost all of us are aware that unpredictable forces are capable of damaging our ability to control movement. We know that when we see a person unable to walk, for example, that we ourselves could be experiencing what we are observing in a heartbeat. Those who sense this connection to a person in a predicament instinctively step in to help someone who is outnumbered. I believe those who do not have this instinct to help may eventually step forward in the future when they make the connection that one day they could have a movement disorder like Parkinson's.

My accounts, many humorous to me in retrospect, are intended to provide an insightful and entertaining look at what happens when one is diagnosed with Parkinson's disease at 54, as I was, and has to learn to deal with an increasingly debilitating physical disorder. This is not a self-help book. Rather, the book is designed to give the reader different frames of reference that could provide insight when dealing with common problems that accompany Parkinson's and other movement disorders. The soul of the book is developed through a series of vignettes based on events I have experienced with Parkinson's disease during the past 16 years.

Some events were life changing, some were just instructive and many, upon reflection, were comic. Often they were defining, prescribing how I viewed myself and the world around me. The experiences added to my understanding of how to cope with Parkinson's. While these observations are unique to me, they have applicability to caregivers and others who are trying to understand Parkinson's or other movement disorders and to those who have these disorders and have experienced what I discuss. (From this point forward, understand when I am referencing PD; those with other movement disorders may have similar experiences.)

PD symptoms have affected my life 24/7 for 16 years. I have had thousands of incidents where Parkinson's impacted me in ways that required a creative response.

These short vignettes help keep the devils of fear and anger at bay and replace them instead with hope and understanding. The conquering of these devils is done by providing a glimpse of the human condition during some of the crazy, unnerving and poignant moments I have experienced because I have Parkinson's, and my body was outnumbered.

Why Me?

My intimate experience with Parkinson's disease began 20 years ago when, at age 74, my father was diagnosed with PD and began his journey dealing with the progress of the disease. I watched him decline from a 6-foot 4-inch healthy senior citizen to a man who was unable to walk without aids. He passed away 16 years ago at age 84. I was diagnosed with Parkinson's within a month of his death. I was 54.

When I was diagnosed with Parkinson's, I was a Professor of Economics and Asian Studies at the University of Montana. Teaching was my passion and my career was on full overdrive with fascinating work just getting underway in emergent China with the U.S. State Department and the Foreign Ministry of China. I also served as an expert witness and economist in civil and criminal litigation, including work for the U.S. Department of Justice, Fortune 500 corporations and public policy litigation.

At the end of my first four years with Parkinson's, I decided to stop teaching because of the inability to manage the side effects of the medication. I couldn't teach without unduly distracting my students and exhausting myself. However, to a person, the undergraduate and graduate students at the University of Montana gave me the most inspiring level of support and genuine accommodation anyone could ever hope for when I was in the classroom.

I was able to keep my expert witness work viable by progressively narrowing its scope until the end of the 10th year. Providing expert testimony requires an extraordinary amount of energy, particularly when preparing for depositions and court room testimony. Eventually, Parkinson's makes testifying in front of judges and juries for long periods of time physically impossible.

I emphasize the continuation of work during the development of Parkinson's to encourage those who eventually face a similar problem to continue working as long as they are very careful to be realistic regarding their changing capacities. In my case, the extraordinary professionalism and ability to look past disability of those working in the federal and state courts throughout the country can never be underestimated.

In general people's capacity to accommodate the presence of disability in everyday life and the workplace can not only be surprising but also, reassuring. And it goes way beyond legal issues of discrimination. Because of the incredible support of others, a person with PD and other chronic physical issues comes to understand why a person is obligated to find the will to fight on and live life to the fullest.

It is my hope that these accounts help develop an understanding of how PD and physical disorders force one into random predicaments. The accounts are chosen to show how people with movement disorders feel outnumbered. For those with Parkinson's, it is important to encourage them to accept the importance of problem solving by accepting the help of others. This book was my way to share the enriching interactions my experience with others has brought me and show how I am able live a full life, "with a little help from my friends."

SECTION 2: DIAGNOSIS

Denial Is Not an Option

Every change in life has a rite of passage associated with the change. When Parkinson's disease has been diagnosed, an affected individual moves into the world of movement disorders.

Parkinson's reveals itself through symptoms. In the beginning, people with Parkinson's often exhibit a tremor. No matter how seemingly trivial the symptom (in my case starting with my left pinky finger) I learned that people will take notice. As a group, people are ever vigilant even when the individual members are not. For example, the Unabomber, living seemingly isolated in the woods of Montana, learned that people not only noticed his presence but also his individual characteristics in some detail, much to his eventual regret.

This story, which I've entitled "The Parky Professor," describes the moment when I had to choose between denial of an obvious physical tremor and dealing with it up front. Denial was not an option. In heeding this lesson I have no regrets and gained considerable unanticipated support. When the symptoms of Parkinson's present themselves, it is clearly better to be open about it than to attempt to cover it up. Denial fools no one but oneself.

Chapter 1
The Parky Professor

The slight shaking in my left pinky finger wouldn't go away. My first inclination was to hide it so that I wouldn't notice it, and perhaps nobody else would either. It turns out that that's absolutely impossible for a professor standing in front of 150 students in a college economics class. A moving pinky finger in a front pocket does not go unnoticed by the conflicted needs of students who want to be educated but actually are desperate to be entertained. The pinky beckons the residual 5-year-old in them all.

It was an interesting moment when I ascertained that I potentially had 300 pairs of eyes watching me, but 217 of them were open and focused squarely on the pinky gyrating in my left pants pocket. Terror struck me. I imagined the males thought of me as a pervert. As for the females, well I have no idea what they thought. I pulled my hand out of the pocket while the pinky waved at the crowd. The students quickly looked down at their notes to check out a legible bit of wisdom they had written down. When they looked up again there was sort of a shuffling, coughing, slightly laughing moment. This was the point where I decided laughter could be a good thing and was the correct path to take.

I could either fake it, pretend that my hand was not shaking, or fess up and deal with the facts of the moment. So I held up the offending hand and said, "Quit that."

It just kept waving.

"This, folks, is Parkinson's," I said "And because I can't control this finger it means I've got it."

Their faces all went blank, which was not uncommon in an economics class, but at least I had changed the subject.

Many years of teaching told me that just facts and terms are not enough. Students need a framework to help them understand where a situation leaves them. An economics class is where students are given a structure to understand economic behavior. At 18 most students have not given critical thought to the structure of the world and, in fact, are focused on exploring their new found independence. Over time the world will give them structure, and they'll find out they are not so independent after all.

So I decided giving them structure to understand this new situation would facilitate the ability to put it in context and understand my ailment.

I needed a way to motivate them to look beyond my waving pinky to retain my teaching effectiveness. I quickly remembered the perfect T-shirt a freshman student once wore. In bold letters the T-shirt said, "I'm Not Yet." Those words gave me a starting point. Thus, I began to try to structure the students' understanding of me as a person. I was also calling on life lessons my daughter taught me in her teenage years. That conversation would go something like this.

I would ask, "What are you doing?"

She would reply, "I'm becoming."

I was always left without anything profound to say, but replied, "Oh, okay."

Those 300 sets of eyes, now very attentive, belonged to

those who were "becoming." I decided to explain.

"Okay, folks, I'm not just trying to be friendly by waving. It turns out that I've just been diagnosed with Parkinson's." Repeating oneself is important in teaching.

There was a mixture of responses.

"Oh, my God."

"What did he say?"

"There's free parking?"

"Will this be on the test?"

Those potentially employable students that pay attention in class folded their arms across their chests, posing a critical stance waiting to see what was going to happen.

"Context, context," flashed in my mind.

"I have the same disease as the Pope, Mohammed Ali and Michael J Fox," I said. "I'm going to shake and exhibit other odd movements and behaviors during this class, so I need to make sure it's not a distraction for you. What you need to remember is that I'm a combination of all these people I just listed, and each personality type appears randomly. So when I'm shaking, remember I have divine inspiration and am infallible; when I freeze in place. I'm the most well-known and toughest guy in the world; and when I drive up in a DeLorean with an old guy as my driver, I'm back to the future, making a sequel to fund research on PD and charming you out of your beer money."

They looked at each other in bewilderment, but with hearty laughs. I saw many accepting nods. We moved on. Whew! With this array of possible ways to define me, I thought we had things covered.

I later learned that they began betting pools on the appearance of symptoms, converting wondering what is going on into a type of asocial behavior that is like betting on the Super Bowl. That's how everyone could participate even though they know nothing about football or Parkinson's. Instead of betting on happenings such as first butt pat, they'd bet on first freeze up on Tuesday; first shaking of both hands on Thursday instead of first hands to the face mask penalty, first stuck behind the podium today instead of first field goal.

For many, the research into things they could bet on with a Parky Professor was their first attempt at online research. So they accidentally achieved one of my academic goals, giving them a feel for applied research and probability theory. In this case they learned more than they intended to, making any professor worth tenure mildly happy. The students were creating order out of chaos.

The more interesting aspects of this situation began to develop very subtly. Students took on self-appointed tasks. For example, when I'd be answering questions after class and look back at a whiteboard I'd used, it would be cleaned. What seemed to come from careful observation or maybe some research on the part of the students was that they realized when I was frozen in front of the class, distraction helped. One of the students away from my field of vision would ask a question. (As Parkinson's people know, as well as observant students, changing the subject tended to unfreeze me.) As soon as the question was asked, I would alter my mental focus to answer it, and then I could move again. The questions were not always perfect, but I don't think that was the point.

If I was particularly "off," some students would make sure I got to my next class or back to my office by walking and talking along with me. When I was fine, or as I say "on," students typically rushed off to their own world. In many ways many of them in turn were covering my back.

My understanding of the complexity of students in this generation was, indeed, changed by their thoughtful, caring and humane reaction to my Parkinson's. In the way they treated me, they demonstrated that though they might be at a point in life where the phrase, "I'm not yet," was appropriate, they definitely were on their way to "becoming."

SECTION 3: UNCHARTED WATERS

Navigating the Healthcare System

Once an individual has passed successfully through denial and faces Parkinson's, a world of institutional structures referred to as the health care system emerges to challenge one's life schedule for time, money and attention. Of course, a person could just go sit in the dark and shake. But as normal individuals, we are unprepared for that option. Most of us are not very good at becoming hermits or constructing psychic caves to live in.

For the non-cave dwelling population with Parkinson's or those who serve as resource people, there is a need to deal with neurologists, medication, physical therapists and psychologists.

Dealing with the mental aspect of Parkinson's can be challenging. It ultimately involves coming to understand the disease. Mind control is a complex process of gaining knowledge and forming attitudes to create a new reality in response to the demands of a chronic disease. The first-order of business is gaining reliable information about Parkinson's. Knowledge impacts choices about neurological care, medication, physical activity and attitude formation. Every decision made in one area, such as medication, impacts choices in all other areas.

In my case, coming to understand Parkinson's became an obsession as I faced a decision about deep brain stimulation (DBS) surgery. It led me to seek input from scientists. For others, the appropriate resources may be psychologists, social workers, family doctors and other health care professionals.

In seeking out information from experts, beware of charlatans. Charlatans can be identified by having a self-declared truth about some aspect of dealing with Parkinson's or other disorders. Their version of truth is likely to make those who listen to them a victim. The charlatan can be identified when they assert that they know what no one else knows without any proof or validation. Charlatans are usually willing to pass their secret unverifiable information on to those who want a quick fix at a special price. They almost always have some sort of paranoid conspiracy, as they describe it, launched against them by people who demand verification. Charlatans most often prey on to people who live in those isolated psychic caves I referred to. They are generally people who desire miracles or easy solutions. To paraphrase a useful rule in science, results that are too good to be true require extraordinary evidence to verify their validity.

Chapter 2
Finding a Neurologist Who Fits: An Odyssey

When the first signs of Parkinson's emerge, denial can occur very easily. In my case the disease presented itself as a tremor of my left little pinky that slowly started to involve the forearm. However, when it is time for an annual physical, the family physician is unlikely to let the patient get away with this blind eye approach to an obvious problem. This is a good thing.

The initial symptoms could, in fact, be a whole host of other conditions from Lou Gehrig's disease to Wilson's disease, conditions that are often catastrophic in fairly short periods of time. Assuming a diagnosis of Parkinson's can lead to serious consequences if the actual condition is determined to be something else. "Don't wait; it'll be too late" is a good phrase to keep in mind.

In my case I was aware that Parkinson's might be the outcome of the diagnosis because my father had died from complications with Parkinson's a month before the PD symptoms appeared in my left hand. What was really unknown was what kind of time frame the progress of Parkinson's would take. In his case, my father began falling due to Parkinson's, but died as a consequence of two failed hip replacements, the side effects of pain management and aging. My family physician recommended that I see a neurologist right away to eliminate the possibility of other explanations and to confirm or reject Parkinson's as a diagnosis. I dutifully scheduled my appointment.

Parkinson's was described to me in many ways but one of the characterizations I heard most often was that everybody's Parkinson's was different. It appeared that PD was fairly unique to the individual even though it involved the same set of symptoms. The variations among people with Parkinson's were in the sequence, the timing and severity of each of the symptoms. This rather unstructured explanation was useful information, but the emphasis on each individual person's experience allowed me to construct a rosy scenario where minor symptoms developed first. In my case a twitching little finger and pin rolling (an involuntary movement of the thumb against the pad of the index finger) were the first symptoms. Since they were not terrifying issues, I went to the neurologist feeling optimistic.

My approach was to show the neurologist how facile I was with my motor skills, even though, based on my father's history, I believed the diagnosis would be Parkinson's. In my fantasy about how the appointment would go, I had the neurologist saying that it would take 50 years to develop. So, at a hundred and four, I could be in trouble. Do you know any people who are hundred and four who are not potentially in trouble? The scene I painted in my mind was uncomfortable but safe territory.

As anyone with PD knows, neurologists go through a standard battery of tests such as touching one's nose, watching the doctor's finger move side to side, walking unaided around in the hall, playing patty cake and enduring pokes to test reflexes. At some point they check the strength of the grip. In my case, this was a big mistake. The neurologist had me grab two fingers on each hand and then said to squeeze hard. I was 6 foot 2 inches, 250 pounds, and I did. His eyes showed a silent scream. "Let me go!" By then I realized that I was showing off, trying to prove to myself that I was okay.

The testing ended immediately. He announced the diagnosis and said that when he had recovered his ability to write, he would forward his notes to my regular physician. I knew he was joking. But I was embarrassed at my behavior, not from anything he did. In fact this doctor cleared up many of my misconceptions. I was fifty-four. I had early-onset Parkinson's that seemed to be progressing fairly quickly. Unfortunately, he was moving on from Montana so I needed to find another neurologist. I didn't realize at the time that this appointment would turn out to be the beginning of an odyssey for me.

In my search for a replacement neurologist I decided to go national. The reason for this was that we had made a commitment as a family to always go to a center of excellence for a second opinion when any one of us faced a serious medical problem. This commitment to a second opinion turned out to be a tremendous asset down the road.

The decision to seek a second opinion took me to Massachusetts General/Harvard, the Mayo Clinic and the University of Southern California. These are amazing professional centers where expertise is concentrated and devoted to research for cures and development of medicines and protocols for the management of Parkinson's and, of course, other diseases as well.

It is almost impossible to believe that they haven't cured this disease because of the collective intelligence and knowledge represented at these and all research centers worldwide. Unfortunately, Parkinson's and other similar diseases are really very difficult to research because there exists no unifying theoretical description of cause and effect.

So far, Parkinson's has frustrated the best minds that are devoted to curing it. Explaining the likelihood for a cure for Parkinson's from research scientists to others leads to a case of what I like to call the "Oxymorons." The possibility of a cure is "hopelessly encouraging," "discouragingly possible," "realistically unlikely," "imminently undeliverable" and on and on. One thing is clear: it is important to think about how to support further research.

In my case it was time to think local as well. At this point we returned home with lots of notes, reports and brain images and a nod of thanks for health insurance coverage.

The next task was to seek a local neurologist who could translate this mass of information into a workable treatment plan. Remember, Parkinson's is an individual experience. This makes the management of medicine extremely difficult. And successful management involves working closely with a neurologist a person can trust. Seeking a compatible neurologist is much like seeking a friend. You need great communication, a shared commitment to common goals and empathy for the other's limitations.

It is difficult to start on a good note with a neurologist because there is no Parkinson's cure. No "we'll fix this" moment occurs. The second limiting factor is that the research has yet to identify exactly what causes Parkinson's. The result is that the neurologist and the patient have to operate within a fairly narrow set of options. There's good news and bad news in this restricted environment. The good news is there are a huge number of medicines that can help with management of Parkinson's symptoms. The bad news is that many of the medicines have very significant side effects. And when or if they work, many times no one knows exactly why.

In my heart of hearts I imagined I would identify with neurologists as a peer economist. Both are intelligent committed professionals dealing with problems (economies) that have no cure, using medicines (policies) where no one knows exactly how or why they work and every patient (citizen) is dealing with a different form or presentation of Parkinson's (economic chaos). In both cases it might be reasonable to ask, "What could go wrong here?"

It turns out a lot can go wrong. In both cases it is important to be careful with expectations. Thinking that neurologists have godlike powers is soon dispelled as they explain what is possible and what is not with regard to treatment. The neurologists I have dealt with were uniformly clear and straight forward regarding the limits of their knowledge and their ability to control the disease.

When I began my search for a local neurologist, I had already been evaluated by six distinctly different ones. My symptoms were moving to bilateral tremors, and I was experiencing the beginning of freezing and stiffness of motion. I was on very low doses of medicine, but I certainly could feel the train coming down the track. When I added up the cumulative advice and commentary from the distinguished group of physicians with whom I had spoken a certain phrase began to emerge: "There's no right neurologist for everyone; success is finding the best personal fit."

The more I thought about this, the more it reminded me of advising young adults about their best choice at the start of a career or about their choice of a college or graduate program. Over the years I have learned that it wasn't the most prestigious company or college that worked out for students, it was the one that fit the person best. In addition, the best fit for me may have to be a series of doctors who changed as symptoms emerged over time. Parkinson's is ever-changing, and though it's a deteriorating situation, it is possible, if not likely, that no one neurologist is going to be the best fit for a person at every stage.

As I continued my odyssey, it was clear that I needed an immediate fix. The symptoms were getting more dramatic, and I was clearly deteriorating. The first neurologist I contacted locally was intense, intelligent and a highly trained specialist in the pharmacology of Parkinson's treatment. This relationship was sort of like a first date with a few dinners to follow. We quickly moved to a strategy where my medicine was tuned to corral my Parkinson's symptoms and stabilize the situation. Unfortunately, this approach comes at a fairly high cost in terms of medicinal side effects. Though my Parkinson's symptoms were somewhat stabilized, the side effects often required detailed discussion to assess. The time required to do this was often in conflict with the schedule of a neurologist who had a huge patient load. This first neurologist was like an emergency room doctor who stabilizes the patient in the short run, depending on later intervention by others. My family and I concluded we should look further.

This essentially meant finding someone who was a neurologist who could manage the medicine and give specific advice on how to manage my lifestyle around Parkinson's. What this meant is that I needed more than a neurologist to help me be deal with such issues as diet, exercise, work load, recreation and day-to-day life. I would not be stretching most people's experience too far to suggest that medical schools do not spend much of their time on these issues as part of a neurologist's training. As a result, the search for a neurologist amounts to finding someone with top-flight training who has a lifestyle similar to that of the patient. With this picture in mind, I was able to find the neurologist who was a good fit for the next stage in taking on Parkinson's.

My next choice was a fly fisherman with a PhD and M.D. who was broadly knowledgeable about the lifestyle problems associated with Parkinson's. Very quickly we were able to move beyond the medication issues to a broader approach. It became apparent, however, that this put an enormous strain on the neurologist. He had a hundred or so clients, and the wear and tear of individualizing his approach to care for each was obviously difficult.

Over time, though I thought I was stabilized, I was deteriorating at a steady rate. He described, and I observed, that many of his patients were in exactly the same situation. He made a tremendous effort, but the cumulative impact of his overall practice was overwhelming him. Ultimately, this led to the closing of his practice. I have been told that high turnover rates in the professions are often linked to the professional trying to sustain what patents value most: availability. The more they become available the more they lose control of time. Unfortunately, the physician's stress begins to escalate the more successful they are.

In the case where a neurologist has restricted availability, it behooves a person with Parkinson's to quickly find a neurologist who is available. The next search was made based on a false premise. The false premise was that I had been pretty stable and, therefore, I needed to relax and find a neurologist who could monitor me and my medicine and just keep me right where I was. Since plateauing is common with Parkinson's, this was logical to me at the time.

While neurologists are well-schooled in Parkinson's treatment, they are not identical in their degree of specialization. Some have extensive experience with Parkinson's, others specialize in closed head injuries and traumatic brain injuries, others specialize in seizure and epilepsy disorders, and the list goes on. It turns out it's very important to screen for these specialties rather than assume there are no differences. All neurologists are not equivalent or nor do they have the same clinical focus or practice. As a result of using too open a screening method, the next neurologist I saw did not specialize in Parkinson's, and I quickly found we were not communicating very well. This was in large part because my Parkinson's was taking on a new stage of complications that took a discerning eye with significant PD background to recognize.

This experience taught me that lack of communication between someone at this stage of progression through

Parkinson's disease and a neophyte neurologist was a bad situation. So I began looking for another neurologist, now certain that my first question would be about their specialization and experience with Parkinson's patients over time. This is not unlike looking for a surgeon to do brain surgery. A surgeon who does a lot of brain surgery and has a very high success rate is preferred to one who does the surgery occasionally, even with good outcomes. It's not that the specific level of skill is different between the surgeons. The key issue is that the doctor who does a great deal of surgery has dealt with a broader range of problems than the occasional practitioner. It is reasonable to expect risk management to be better with more experience than with less.

Having honed my search skills, I was able to find a Parkinson's specialist who had used her understanding to develop high level listening skills and a very subtle eye for changes in Parkinson's symptoms. Her skills and her knowledge allowed for good communication and a fine tuned matching of medicine to handle the subtle changes in my Parkinson's condition.

I ended my odyssey with a very good fit for my needs, and I learned a great deal from each neurologist along the way. This odyssey emphasizes that finding the right fit involves taking it one step at a time. The question that remains for every degenerative disease seems to be, "How many more steps will I be taking?" Whatever that progression becomes, I felt this neurologist would recognize the changes and communicate with me. She had no plans to leave town, but in medicine there are never guarantees.

Chapter 3
Medicine: Wild Thing

Some years ago I was in a group of parents gathered at a summer lake party when a bright, handsome young man in a shy, but offhanded voice asked a beautiful young woman, somewhat older than he was, if she would like to take a ride on the lake in his boat.

She smiled, perhaps knowing how brave he was to put his ego on the line, and asked, "Why not? I'll meet you at the dock."

The young man changed color; he seemed suddenly out of breath and whirled around. "I'll get the boat ready." he said

A few minutes later, to the putt-putt little roar of a motorboat engine, a 14-foot, shiny aluminum boat pulled out of the dock. The vision was striking: an earnest young man at the helm and a beautiful young, but sophisticated woman holding her broad brimmed hat sitting in the bow as the boat pulled out onto the lake. On its port side one could not miss reading its name, Wild Thing.

Today, wild thing represents something very different to me than hoping a pretty girl will answer yes to a boat ride.

It represents the high hopes of first infatuation with a drug and the unexpected, but inevitable, disappointment that comes with experience.

This scene reminds me of a typical PD person's experience with medicine: It isn't always what it seems to be. Early in the disease a person fantasizes and imagines that medication will do wonders, just like lovers only see each other's good qualities in the beginning of a romantic relationship.

Then reality sets in. Even if the medicine works as promised, side effects beyond what one expects — despite pages of warnings — very frequently present themselves. What's even more disheartening is that if the medication doesn't work, those nasty side effects may still occur. Taking a new "miracle" drug becomes more and more disturbing with each trial. Keeping hope alive, without becoming cynical about medication efficacy, becomes harder over time. More often than not, even if it works for a while, medicine that was once a friend ends up as an adversary.

Prescription medication is as much a part of dealing with Parkinson's as pain is a part of boxing; it comes with the territory. Medication for Parkinson's attempts to deal with the symptoms of a disease whose cause is not well understood by the most well-trained, brightest and most creative scientists in our society. Unfortunately, the final result of the best science currently available is a very small pill. Sometimes it is a patch. The pill or patch embodies only a small portion of the scientific effort and is a compromise between what the science is seeking to understand and the necessity to produce something that works now.

The pill is given to someone who really has no idea what taking it will do to them. Yet, because of the science behind the medication and the clinical testing, it does offer hope that it will fix a symptom such as a tremor or the inability to initiate walking. The motivation to take the medicine is powerful. This combination of high hopes and potential significant disappointment means that taking medicine is the start of a person's relationship with the "wild thing."

Trying to use medication to fight the symptoms of Parkinson's disease is a delicate balancing act. Because there is no cure for Parkinson's, not only are neurologists unable to take the "we'll fix this" approach to overall medical care, they also face tremendous uncertainty when prescribing medication. By this I mean there is currently no medicine that will prevent PD's progress as a degenerative condition. In some cases science does not know how or why a specific medicine is effective. No matter how successful the medicine is at any one point, when symptoms change, what worked yesterday might not work tomorrow.

Because I am not an expert in the field of pharmacology, I can't give advice on what medicine works and what doesn't. A writer without unlimited errors and omissions insurance should not play pharmacist. I am only relating to the reader what happened to me as I took various medications over the past fifteen years. That is why in this chapter I gave each medication I took an invented, behavioral name. This transfers the emphasis from the medication to the effect it had on me. Not everyone, of course, will experience the same outcomes even with the same medications. Taking almost any medication to deal with Parkinson's has always been an experience similar to following Alice in Wonderland down the rabbit hole. That's why I describe all of the medications I have taken grouped together as the "***wild thing***."

"Old Person"

The first medicine I was prescribed to help with PD I called "Old Person," because it has been around for many years. I don't know whether it could have worked when I first took it, because I was nauseous within a very short period after ingesting it. I couldn't hang with "Old Person" more than a few days.

"Fire in the Pants" and "Sleeps While Awake": the Pills

The next medications prescribed were a new drug and its older ally formed into a dynamic cocktail. I called the drugs "Fire in the Pants" and "Sleeps While Awake." The combination slowed down my tremor by about 50 percent which was just enough to allow me get to bed in anticipation of two days of the full effect, which consisted mostly of side effects. "Fire in the Pants" felt like injecting cayenne pepper between bones in the lower spine, like a saddle block given to women during or after birth. Instead of the lower half of the body going numb, "Fire in the Pants" caused my nerves to ignite in a firestorm that was truly astonishing.

At the same time "Sleeps While Awake" put my mind into a state of awareness that I believe is similar to the one experienced just before a driver falls asleep at the wheel. The difference is no sleep occurs, no jolting drop of the head, rather just a dulling of the senses. It did, however reduce Parkinson's tremors substantially.

Clearly this trade-off was not acceptable. I, of course, stopped taking the cocktail and dealt with the shakes, feeling slightly more kinship toward the rhythm of my own tremors than the trauma of the mind dulling "Sleeps While Awake" medication. It would have been impossible for me to tolerate for one more second the excruciating pain from "Fire in the Pants."

My neurologist shook his head at my story, observing he sort of expected the sleepy effects but that the fire in the legs problem was pretty rare. We decided to look elsewhere.

"Travels with Little Friend"

The next medication involved the medicine I called,

"Travels with Little Friend." This next medication was an attempt to utilize a relatively new concoction recently out of clinical trials which was designed to work by acting in place of dopamine, a natural substance in the brain needed to control movement. I think it achieved that objective because my tremors became less pronounced, my "off" periods were less severe, particularly the stiffness, and freezing problems abated somewhat.

The tricky part was that I began hallucinating. At first it was very subtle. But as time moved on and the dosage increased, the hallucination became much clearer. In my case the specific illusion was a new companion. So, whenever I met anybody it became a threesome. I never made introductions. But it was a bizarre experience as I managed the effects of "Travels with Little Friend." I really didn't know what to do because my little friend would come and go, and never seemed to want to do anything in particular. After a short while, I began to think how awkward it would be if my little friend decided to have its own personality. Going back to the doctor seemed the logical course of action. The neurologist confirmed that hallucinations do sometimes accompany this medication, as he had initially warned me. I remembered that. But since I'd never discussed any ground rules with my little friend, I suggested ending the friendship. I needed to try a different medication. The neurologist agreed.

"Sleeps While Awake": the Patch

The next medication was selected because of the increasing variability of my symptoms. The "on" and "off" cycles were getting more extreme. The approach was to try out a patch of "Sleeps While Awake" where the dosage could be made level 24 hours a day, eliminating cyclical effects caused by taking pills at intervals throughout the day. "Fire in the Pants" was not considered again.

At first the patch of "Sleeps While Awake" seemed to work very well on the tremors and other Parkinson's symptoms, so there were good results for a while. However, as the medicine reached the targeted level, the narcoleptic problem returned with no variation during the day or night. Meaning, I never really was awake and never really asleep throughout a 24-hour period. After about three days, it was clear that my mind could not tolerate this condition despite the improvement in my symptoms.

The other problem with the patch was that even after it reached a target level in the system, the medicine remained in the system for a while even after discontinued.

When I had been evaluated at Massachusetts General Hospital/Harvard, the neurologist expressed his general concern about the trend toward medicines taken once or twice a year having side effects that, even when the medicine was stopped, would continue for six months or more. For the four days after I removed the "Sleeps While Awake" patch I thought about him frequently. It took that long for me to get back to my normal tremors and symptoms. Imagine waiting six months for that to happen? Getting my symptoms back and sleeping was comforting, much to my dismay.

The patch also had a very significant danger associated with its use. If it fell off, no one should touch it but me. This threat existed because the person picking it up might accidently get a dose of the medication. That experience could be potentially dangerous, since an unsuspecting person would have too much dopamine in his or her system to handle. This problem was especially disconcerting for me since I often have young grandchildren running around in their normal curious state.

"Spinning Eagles"

The next round of attempts to prescribe medication that

would work on my PD involved trying out a number of relatively new medicines that seemed to have no effect on my tremors or other Parkinson's symptoms. They had virtually no side effects either. Nothing ventured, nothing gained. The result was discouraging because the list of potential medications was shrinking rapidly. I labeled this group of pills "Spinning Eagles," a backhanded compliment for a big deal that doesn't go anywhere.

"Old Person" Plus Anti-Nausea Pills

At this point, I had gone through some 10 medications and five or six neurologists. I had lots of experience with drugs and few options left. Very cleverly, my neurologist suggested we try "Old Person" another time, only in combination with an anti-nausea medication for this experiment. This suggestion was impressive, in part because the neurologist had taken the time to go back through my now enormous file in detail. As with any good detective, he found a lead that had not been followed up on in the past.

This combination of drugs turned out to be a very successful strategy. I only needed the anti-nausea medicine for a week or so and my body adapted to the presence of "Old Person." My tremor became significantly diminished, and my symptoms when I was "on" were virtually nonexistent. When I was "off," they were diminished. The downside of this medication was that research showed it stopped working after seven to 10 years, depending on the person taking it. This makes it a very difficult choice for young onset Parkinson's patients. If one starts this medicine at 35, it may stop working at 45. With life expectancy at about 78 to 80 years across genders in the U.S. this issue is problematic to say the least. With this medication a person gets to choose when he will have no access to a medication that works. As a result, many people hold off beginning a relationship with "Old Person" for as long as possible.

The other problem with "Old Person" is that over time dosage must increase to deliver the same effectiveness. Increasing the amount of the medication in the system creates a problem called dyskinesia which is induced by the medicine itself. As those with PD know, dyskinesia is commonly a jerky, dance-like movement of the arms and/or head and upper torso. This seems to transform "Old Person" into "Dances with Old Person." However, it does transform an "off" time when I can hardly walk to a time when I can walk while gyrating like one of those, blower driven, 15-foot-tall Gumby-like monstrosities by the road which are used to beckon customers to get gas, get an oil change, even buy a car. This option, when the time comes, is not easy, but is one of the now narrowing set of options for a long term patient with PD. At least with this situation, I was not frozen in place. The solution was combining this medicine with a long acting medication I called, "Strolling with Old Person" which has given me seven to eight years of relative stability out of the last 15.

Accurate predictions are notoriously hard to make with PD. Unfortunately, the one about "Old Person" losing its potency came true as predicted. Its effectiveness ended abruptly. This situation was much worse than expected because the gap between the medicine working effectively and the baseline level of Parkinson's symptoms without "Old Person" had widened enormously over the seven to eight year period. In fact the problem was sufficient to make me begin to look at options that might reduce medicine dependency such as deep brain stimulation (DBS).

DBS is a much discussed brain surgery technique that potentially has big rewards associated with it. There are some risks associated with the procedure. It also requires regular maintenance and fine tuning, at least with the current system of electrodes inserted deep in the brain. No matter what it is called, as one neurologist reminded me, "It's brain surgery!"

"Flying No Feathers" and "Long Runner Old Person"

My first response was to question my neurologist about any medications that could postpone DBS to the distant future. She responded by aggressively seeking a combo that might work for a while and in a month or so found me a new cocktail. It consisted of some new friends whose names I dubbed "Long Runner Old Person" and "Flying No Feathers." "Long Runner Old Person" was a newly developed long-acting "Old Person" that had been recently made available. "Flying No Feathers" was a medicine that worked to subdue Parkinson's symptoms, although scientists have only a vague idea why it helps. It was originally developed to deal with another disease.

I will end the discussion of the crooked and bumpy trail which I have traveled through the land of pills and patches with a note about trying out a medication when its functionality isn't understood. I fondly called this drug "Flying No Feathers" because it was in keeping with my previous experience with the "wild thing" of PD medication effects.

"Flying No Feathers" works to subdue Parkinson's symptoms and supports the "on" state for people with the disease.

If a person is "on" due to taking "Flying No Feathers," that person may be "flying" along nicely. Since neither the person nor the scientists understand fully what causes the medicine to work, there is no way of knowing what to do when the medicine stops working. When a medicine stops working, it leaves a person extremely vulnerable. I imagined as I looked for a name, the situation would be like a bird soaring on high suddenly losing all of its feathers. What should a person do? Take more medicine? Get a different doctor? The person might assume a new medicine will be available very quickly, before they crash. This is extremely unlikely.

The shortcomings of medications are related to the fact that we have yet to determine the ultimate cause or find a cure for Parkinson's. The fundamental solution to this problem is research. Until research solves these fundamental issues, medication is the main weapon in our arsenal at any given time. No pill or patch can perform beyond the knowledge gleaned from research and evidence from clinical trials. Research allows us to know which action will impact the physical and cognitive issues we face as we deal with Parkinson's. New research findings will be the only and most reliable way to tame the "wild thing."

Chapter 4
Physical Therapy:
A Creative Art

After being diagnosed with Parkinson's, I decided that it was important to develop a positive and well-directed program of exercise and competitive sports to retain my hand-eye coordination, balance and agility, let alone keep myself in shape and have some fun while doing it. What surprised me was that Parkinson's tended to blindside me. I had visions of having my own personal trainer. Instead I got a physical therapist. In an insidious way, Parkinson's progression tends to unbalance the body both structurally and chemically, leading to unforeseen problems.

As I continued to upgrade my exercise through more weightlifting and bicycle riding and playing handball, I thought I could come close to the conditioning I had in my thirties.

No matter how much exercise I did, I spent more time walking than exercising. It was the walking that got me. My Parkinson's progressed from the left arm downward into the left leg, and without paying a lot of attention to this progression I began to alter my stride. At first, I was just trying to step forward with the left leg since it seemed to fall behind the right. Next, I began rotating on the right leg through the knee up to the hip to compensate for the left leg limp. This had the effect of reducing the harm limping caused to the left leg, but it caused increased pain to the right hip and right knee. Ironically, the more exercise I did, the more my gate seemed to worsen. So instead of a great bicycle ride on a beautiful sunny day through Montana, I found myself at the orthopedic surgeon's office.

Frankly, I didn't like the reality I had to hear from the orthopedic surgeon. Since my right knee had been operated on 35 years earlier for ACL and MCL damage as well as a torn meniscus, my little adjustment to the limp had brought me bone on bone grinding and a baker's cyst full of fluid behind my knee. The answer to my problem was for me to lose 30 pounds, go to physical therapy and learn how to walk properly. If this were not successful, a total knee replacement was in order. The entire burden was on me. This was turning out to be serious. I have never dieted and to me, at that time, PT seemed even unlikely to work. Still I had little choice but to try.

PT and half rations were not exactly what I imagined as I headed into retirement. My immediate answer was to start eating one half of what I normally ate. Surprise, I started losing weight. This was not complicated. I now ate fewer calories than I used.

The other directive was to go to physical therapy which meant I had to forego at least some other exercise I enjoyed. I went to physical therapy.

Surprisingly, the first session started with what might be described as wimpy exercises at weight levels that are almost embarrassing for a full grown man. The next thing the PT prescribed was movement exercises that were so easy there seemed to be no possible gain from this activity.

I got a nod and smile from the therapist when I

protested. "These exercises don't seem hard enough to have an effect." Within 15 minutes I was exhausted from doing the next set of little exercises requested by my 102-pound physical therapist. Now out of breath, I asked her what she was going to accomplish with this particular exercise.

"I'm going to kill you," she said sarcastically, and then laughed.

I tried to laugh, and I knew at that point I had the right physical therapist.

She proceeded to show me exercises for body parts I didn't know I had. The one I can describe the best is where the patient lies flat on his or her back and throws one leg over the other while twisting the torso the other direction. Then he or she lifts the thrown leg skyward slowly against pressure. Over time this form of torture strengthens muscles which help to stabilize the connection between the back and the gluteus through the hip. This process was part of overcoming the damage I was doing compensating for the limp brought on by Parkinson's. It worked. It turned out that my physical therapist had special knowledge of the muscles that I had failed to exercise with my other physical activities.

Three months later, having lost 35 pounds, I returned, walking properly, to the orthopedic surgeon. He inspected me, checked my weight and looked up saying in the best southern drawl he had, "Nobody does that."

"Didn't I tell you I really hate surgery?" I asked.

He observed that somebody who probably hated surgery just as much as I did but couldn't stop eating anyway would take my slot in surgery. I observed that too little credit was given to the physical therapist.

"I know her, she'll kill you."

"Almost," was my reply.

Over the years my Parkinson's developed, and I have continued to exercise and play a competitive sport when I could. However, the progress of Parkinson's destabilized my body in numerous ways. One of the most obvious, and certain to be common among people with Parkinson's, is the effect of being frozen in place while sleeping. With PD the body fails to move while asleep. Tremors usually abate during REM sleep, but hours can elapse between rolling over and stretching. In my case, the primary effect was to constantly cause pressure on my shoulder nerves, creating pain that extended down the arms through the back.

The PT program of exercise and vigorous workouts helped my strength and agility, but was eventually overwhelmed by the Parkinson's progression. However, in every stage physical therapy helped me manage the problem. This involved constantly making adjustments to my physical therapy program so that I could manage my body at a reduced level of activity without pain. I have always been astonished at how creative the therapists were.

Maintaining my body involved the constant search for a physical therapist who had experience with Parkinson's patients. Eventually, the aging process, along with Parkinson's, reduces agility and balance. With me it began to undermine my ability to play handball. I can distinctly recall one of my physical therapists interrupting my comments about how frustrating a particular exercise was by pointing out that I needed to realize having Parkinson's does not mean the aging process stops. She was working on "getting old" issues with the exercise. That was a healthy reminder that everything that happens to people physically when they have PD is not always due to Parkinson's. That reminder is very instructive to remember.

In dealing with the problem of loss of balance and agility, my PT team was wonderfully creative. A serious problem arose because I started falling down when I tangled up my legs backing up. This was bad for me when playing handball, and it was not good for the other three guys on the court when we played doubles.

At that point, I had a team of two physical therapists putting their heads together to work on my problems. One was the analyst who kept using all the data she had collected in my various tests of agility endurance and range of motion. The second therapist used that information and adapted certain exercises to attack the problem.

This process involved a progression of planned workouts from walking forward and backward on elevated tubes while playing catch to moving back and forth over taped patterns on the floor while playing catch with a weighted medicine ball. And finally being hooked to the wall with bungee cords that provided resistance and performing modified basketball drills until both the physical therapist and I were exhausted. Other people in physical therapy began to take note of this unusual therapy activity. One day we reached the point where everyone, including all the physical therapists in the entire facility, stopped what they were doing to watch the PT work with me.

My physical therapist brought in his boxing gloves and padded hand guards and then put tape on the floor to make sure I didn't cross my legs. Then we began boxing. I overheard comments such as, "I never saw that before at physical therapy;" "I don't think I can do that;" "What does that fix?" The place became much more interesting and fun as a result of our new regimen to attack my Parkinson's.

Most importantly, it worked. I was able to play handball for a while longer without falling down because I had practiced boxing. Survival in boxing necessitates backing up while keeping the feet apart and not crossing one's legs. These are essential elements in avoiding getting knocked out. My PT was responsible for designing a very creative solution to my problem that wasn't in the least bit wimpy.

Chapter 5
"The RGS4 Protein Needs Dopamine or Parkinson's Occurs"

"The RGS4 Protein Needs Dopamine or Parkinson's Occurs."
   I read this recently out loud to myself from an article my son-in-law sent me from Italy: the RGS4 protein needs dopamine or Parkinson's occurs. My mind whirled with a couple of questions. First of all, what did this mean? Second of all, was this an important finding or not?
   Thinking along these lines for the umpteenth time reminded me that many people are caught between two types of information. The first is found in materials such as books, pseudo-scientific summary articles for the lay public and internet blogs without much depth which are easy to read. The second is real science material written for the scientific and medical community which most people can't read and understand.
   I was one of those people who didn't understand this scientific article.
   I have a PhD in economics which is accompanied by a

working knowledge of statistics and mathematics, as well as years of working professionally as an expert witness with psychologists, engineers and even chemists. Yet articles in biochemistry, physiology, neurology and neuropsychology are very difficult, if not impossible, for me to decipher. But I do know enough to be suspicious of drug company claims and articles in a variety of places which seem to announce big discoveries or hopeful studies relating to curing PD or offering to control symptoms. The reason for the skepticism was my father's experience over the 20 years from his diagnosis of Parkinson's where no break-through cures actually materialized. During this period many studies seem to suggest that miracles were just around the corner.

This would not matter so much if many of us didn't have to make very important decisions that would be enormously enhanced if a person knew how to judge the efficacy of information available. Many of us are stranded somewhere between popular press promises and scientific information we cannot interpret. A typical scenario might be demonstrated by the following experience.

While I was whirling around the room experiencing another episode of being overdosed and having dyskinesia caused by my medication, I said to myself, "I would like some information about my realistic options." The answer to this question involved knowing which drugs were in the pipeline, their potential capacity and availability to fix this problem verses brain surgery, a difficult to reverse procedure.

The onset of dyskinesia meant that my meds were not going to work well, or at all, anymore, and I'd be forced to consider deep brain stimulation (DBS) surgery. My reaction was, no matter what it's called, it is brain surgery. This would be a consequential action, and I had to make an informed decision.

I usually evaluate big decisions in a conversation with my dog Piper, a chow Border collie mix. She allow one sided conversations. All final decisions are made with my wife; they are decidedly not one sided.

"Insanity is often defined as doing the same thing over and over and expecting different results each time," I blurted to the dog on this occasion. I added, "I've taken every medication available, and the side effects are too strong or they don't work." In exasperation I announced, "I would be insane to wait for a new medication; let's do the DBS."

Saying this aloud made me even more unsettled.

The dog just sat down and rolled over looking for a belly-rub, no doubt thinking that's what I'd said.

She got what she wanted as I sought clarity. "When I am spinning around the room, it is time to do something other than appear like someone acting crazy. Do I take the risk of DBS or bet on a new drug developed out of the research on dopamine derived from the analysis in the article?"

"Think outside the box," I mumbled. I made sure not to say this too loud because what I didn't need was the dog to start spinning around the room with me. So I decided to think outside the box and get more and better first-hand information rather than that filtered through the health care system.

A university setting is outside the box for most people, but not me. I searched the University of Montana website for a biochemist who might translate the protein article. I found not only a biochemist, but one whose specialty was G proteins. Amazing! After examining his various titles, it was clear this was my man.

I sent him an email asking if, over a beer, he might help me decipher the article I was reading and the scientific article it principally relied on. "If you don't ask, there is no chance to learn," I mumbled to myself. I reasoned that I might re-contact him again in a week.

In about fifteen minutes I get a reply that said, "Sure, I will look into it, and I'll get back to you on that beer offer."

Within a couple of days, I received a detailed evaluation of the articles and the suggestion that not only was the subject interesting, but furthermore, that he needed to contact a neurophysiologist to check out his interpretation of the article.

When I got to my book group that afternoon. I mentioned how impressed I was with this professor's response during the pre-literary small talk. One of my colleagues said, "That's an interesting question you've asked him. You know I'm a physiologist. Send me the articles and this fellow's comments, and I'll take a look at them."

By Monday of the following week we scheduled a get together where the three of us could sit down and make sense of this article and others they'd recommended. The timing could not have been better. I was in Stage II of DBS evaluation and just about to meet with the neuropsychologist to find if I were still a good candidate. Stage I was an evaluation by a neurosurgeon who reviewed my enhanced brain scan. I had been designated a good candidate in Stage I. Stage III would be brain surgery should I decide to commit to it.

Sparing the details of the discussion that took place among the scientists and me, the outcome was that the current protein research related to the problems I was having. The follow-up to the research was going to be a clinical evaluation combined with other clinical trials on related research and emerging medicines. This new information suggested to me that I should wait as long as possible to have DBS. Of course, this was a stretch. Yet, now I had new information to make an educated decision.

I met with the neuropsychologist who'd evaluated my neuropsychological test results, and he informed me that I was a very good candidate for DBS. Based on the discussion I had with the scientists, I was able to ask very pointed questions which the neuropsychologist answered in great detail. I told him my decision for the time being. He supported that decision at the time. It is hard to describe how thankful I was for the two scientists who had helped me make a decision by sharing their knowledge with me in a language that made sense.

I was at least in a comfort zone. Yet, my comfort zone was not bounded by what I call smiling-nod ignorance, but by key markers to look for that might change my decision. Smiling-nod ignorance (SNI) is a term I use to describe those instances where a person is listening to something they don't understand, yet they smile and nod as though they do. It is very dangerous to make important decisions when a lack of knowledge causes smiling and nodding rather than curiosity in dealing with experts. It is unclear that anyone is served well when someone is trying to learn is smiling and nodding, and an expert is trying to explain a concept.

I had been an economics professor for 35 years, and as might be imagined, I saw SNI an unbelievable number of times. It always made me uncomfortable. A professor's job is to cure SNI. My experience reading about new discoveries and Parkinson's has made the company of scientists more and more important to me. All I had to do was ask. I learned they are also willing to meet in bars and share information over a beer. In my case I've discovered imported non-alcoholic beer. Alcohol tends to interfere with my medications and make me groggy. Groggy is not a condition you want be in when talking to scientists about your decision whether or not to have brain surgery.

SECTION 4: PREDICAMENTS

The Outside World Forces Your Hand

Who's in Charge Here?

Parkinson's is a neurodegenerative disease that might be better labeled a condition. Commonly, the term disease has a communicable aspect. PD is not communicable except possibly in a rather roundabout way through inherited genetic characteristics. Inheriting Parkinson's per se has not been fully understood, though there appear to be many indicators suggesting that at least a genetic propensity may exist. Eventually, Parkinson's may be identified through genes associated with its existence. No matter what explains how Parkinson's is caused, the eventual deterioration of physical and/or cognitive skills can lead to individuals being classifiable as disabled.

Being in a special class, such as disabled, can prove a great asset or a substantial impediment to freedom of action. The following two accounts show how being "special," or disabled, can complicate dealing with such large organizations as airlines. An individual effort to control a situation while being disabled leads occasionally to winding up in a predicament that provides complex problem solving challenges.

My experience with airlines has been very memorable, though dealing with public services, large retailers and contractors, can also make a person wonder who's in charge. Though disabled people are supposed to be a protected special class, sometimes the effect is like an innocent person of interest caught in a bizarre investigation of why they think they're special.

It is important to remember that agencies, airlines and corporations are not living things. They are just the person you're dealing with at any moment. That is a very good starting point.

Airlines

Airlines have unique characteristics and powers and tend to consider their status special as well. For people who have specific limits on their capacity to function within the unique environment created by the airline, airline operations are often very difficult to manage.

When boarding an airplane, you should anticipate moments when your individual needs confront security issues and the established routines of airline and airport personnel, from ticketing to getting baggage and going home. By asking for accommodation you are taking these people, who are supposed to serve, into uncharted territory. You need a tactic to take charge of defining the problem.

Define the problem so that it is a third, fairly neutral, aspect of the situation. Make the solution easy for them and discuss the impact beyond yourself. Link your issue to consequences they want to avoid, such as crowding of aisles, calling on airplane personnel multiple times, conflict with other passengers, delaying on-time departures, safety issues and going over their head to a manager. This prior proper planning is easier as you become more experienced, which means you have to take the risk involved with being out and active.

For some, not planning ahead complicates the situation so much that staying home almost becomes a refuge. The problems of being out and about should not outweigh the advantages. Changing the balance in favor of the advantages requires perseverance and flexible responses to real people. I have had modest success in exercising my right to be an active person in the world through planning. I learned I had to stay in control, be well informed and charge ahead in spite of having to deal with narrowly focused people.

Chapter 6
"Oh, I Know Someone with Parkinson's"

"Oh, I know someone with Parkinson's."

Hearing this line creates one of those moments where I know I'm about to find out if the airline representative is about to do something to make the situation worse or solve my problem in a thoughtful way. Their next statement will clearly inform me regarding which fork in the road I am on.

In this case, she went on to state, "The extra time should be no problem for you." It was clear I was about to be done in by someone who was going to define my problem for me. What I wanted to hear was, "Could you please tell me what impact the changes in your flight itinerary are going to have on your disability?" thus signaling that the person was going to work with me to solve the problem.

I was rebooking existing airline reservations because the airline had changed the second leg. The final flight on a long trip now increased a layover at an intermediate destination from three to seven hours and delayed my final destination arrival time by 20 minutes. This pushed my arrival time beyond midnight in the middle of winter in Montana. This later flight was frequently canceled at the last moment. The earlier flight from the intermediate stop departed before my now delayed arrival. This change required me to manage seven hours in the layover airport with a high probability of the final flight leg being cancelled. This unilateral move on the part of the airline on an existing reservation seemed like just another annoyance in what I've come to call travel land. This is a place where humans are cargo and revenue units, not people anymore. The airline had apparently explored no other options.

The one hour phone call to resolve the problem created by this combination of poor people management and logistics is the type of ordinary event that becomes complex when faced by someone with Parkinson's.

The problem arises from the fact that Parkinson's is a condition where you are "on" sometimes and "off" at other times. In my case, the "off" state for Parkinson's is one where I move very slowly, freeze up and am stiff and hardly able to walk while experiencing noticeable hand tremors. The "on" state for many people with Parkinson's, including myself, is a time when I am able to move fairly normally, the tremor is hardly noticeable, and while I'm stiff, it's not too far from the creakiness that often occurs with aging. In most cases, the difference between the "on" and "off" period is the efficacy of the Parkinson's medicine at that time.

As a result of this switching from one state to another, some people who think they understand Parkinson's, view it from their past experience with the "on" period, and believe that the "off" situation is potentially fake; or that being "off" exists because of some mistake on the patient's part, such as not taking meds properly or not being tough enough to manage the problems. It is unclear whether these people come to this conclusion because that's the experience they have had with people they actually know who have

Parkinson's, or whether it is based on their general world view that people should just buck up and push through a problem. They do not understand that willpower cannot conquer a basic failure of body chemistry.

The alternative scenario is composed of those who come to understand that the Parkinson's default is "off." Being "on" is a blessing resulting from the proper use of medication, getting good sleep, avoiding stress, being engaged in healthful exercise and finding some magical alignment of the stars and the body's metabolism. With all of these variables, being able to control the timing of being "on" as Parkinson's progresses is increasingly unpredictable and difficult.

In the hour on the phone trying to resolve the delayed flight problem with the airline, I wound up dealing with people who had different perceptions regarding PD.

When the voice on the other end of the phone said, "Those 20 extra minutes should be no problem for you," I suggested that we needed to work on a reservation change and that her attempt at diagnosing my capacities was inappropriate. I thought this was a well-intentioned attempt to stay on task in the negotiation. She obviously didn't agree.

A condescending voice retorted, "I'm not playing doctor. You now have seven hours to get ready for a flight that arrives 20 minutes later than the one you had before."

It made no sense for her to focus on the 20-minute delayed arrival when my problem was with the seven-hour layover and the probable cancellation of the last flight home. I was focused entirely on the problem of dealing with the seven hours of medication management and the potential cancellation, not the 20 minutes of extra travel she was insisting was the point of reference. It was clear to me that she was going to be unrelenting with her point of view. In part to test that hypothesis I responded, "We will take a flight the next day."

"That change will cost you under our rules," she replied.

Hypothesis confirmed!

"You mean there are no alternatives?" I asked.

The response was no longer remotely friendly, but now intentionally officious. She blurted out, "You can pay the change fee plus the additional airfare charges for you and your wife."

"You mean there's nothing we can do about my being dropped in Denver due to a schedule change by the airline at one o'clock in the afternoon and not being able to get to Montana until midnight without paying an extra sum of money when there are flights the next morning?"

"No. I'll check with my supervisor on the cost to you and your wife." Click!

Suddenly I was on hold listening to that numbing music that once took you up, up and away to dreamy places in comfort. After about three minutes of listening to this horrid music blaring out of the cheap speaker on the phone at too loud an amplitude, causing feedback and bizarre tonal shifts, I reached to switch off the speaker.

I was on speaker because my hands sometimes shake so badly that I wind up talking while banging the phone against my head. Trying to switch the speaker off is tricky with a trembling hand. In this case I cut the connection. Yes, there is a magical combination of keystrokes that invariably only a trembling hand can activate. This combination always leads to cutting off phone calls. How did the designer of the phone overlook this problem? How is the call deactivated according to the manual? Where is the manual?

I stared at the silent phone.

Now what? I could just lick my wounds, taking some blame that I didn't handle that very well and accept my fate at the hands of some airline efficiency programmer who is likely controlling policy by maximizing revenue based on a pricing system designed by an economist. I'm an economist. Now I was a victim of my own science. I would not accept this situation!

Tremor in check for a moment, I redialed the airline knowing that I'm playing Russian roulette with my reservation. The nature of the next airline representative was at best a random draw.

I, of course, got a different person. So we had to go through the whole story all over again. After pointing out the change in my reservation I heard the following, "I notice you have requested wheelchair assistance between your flights. Is that correct?"

"Yes, I have Parkinson's and can clearly have mobility problems depending on how I'm doing at the time."

"I see. I have a neighbor who is wheelchair-bound sometimes, and his friends take him fishing which often means they have to pick him up and put him in a seatbelt equipped chair in the boat. He loves to fish. I've often wondered if he has Parkinson's."

I froze. At that moment I had no idea which fork in the road we were about to take. Was this person going to view things from the "on" perspective or the "off" perspective? That was the question of the moment.

The airline representative's tone softened, and she said, "How can I help you with your problem? It looks like you have a seven-hour break between flights and a midnight arrival in Missoula after starting that morning in Costa Rica at 7:30 a.m. Whew, that's exhausting to even think about."

The air quietly flowed out of my lungs, and I said, "I'm unsure whether I can really manage that situation."

"Let's see what we can do."

Hurrah, she was going to let me evaluate my situation and help in whatever way she could. She was going to treat me as though my default situation was "off." She was protecting me from the downside risk rather than forcing me to overcome the problem by assuming the upside is attainable with some certainty through my efforts.

In the end this helpful woman represented the airline very well and within the rules arranged for us to fly out the next day with no extra airline charges. We only had to pay for our lodging. Amazingly, during the course of this exchange, the first representative interrupted us and complained that I cut her off, and we should be charged $500 each for the change fee and change in ticket price. The second representative was extremely helpful and discussed the situation with her supervisor who didn't apply the fee or change in ticket price costs on us. The problem of a likely cancellation became moot. The airline now had a customer for the long-term.

The difference between the two representatives seemed to be based on their differing personal interpretation of Parkinson's. The first focused solely on the 20 minutes extra travel time, and the second listened to me explain the problems of being stuck in an airport for seven hours with uncertainty. The first one felt because the change was trivial to her, she remained in control. The second recognized that the dramatic change in schedule and risk of cancellation meant that I was in the best position to judge how that could be managed.

Disability is psychologically difficult, particularly where uncertainty is a factor. It becomes even more problematic when a person has to convince someone that the disability is real and impacted by circumstance. Parkinson's frequently causes this kind of discrepancy in treatment by people who have seen it, but do not understand that it has a very different presentation from hour to hour and day to day.

Even people with Parkinson's have choices. Too bad it can't be when or how long to be "on" or "off." As part of my planning, I need to know the rules for schedule changes in addition to knowledge of alternative airlines' schedules when I travel.

Chapter 7
"We Don't Give Out Blankets Anymore."

I always set up wheelchair assistance whenever I fly, especially when I have to make connections. I never know if I will go from an "on" to an "off" state over the course of a trip. I hate this unpredictability and so does my wife. We have become careful to take very little luggage on the plane and check as few things as possible so that if I'm out of commission, she doesn't wind up looking like a Sherpa tangled in bags thrashing around the airport. In addition, I start getting ready about 48 hours before any flight. I space out my meds to make sure that I start the trip "on." I also try to get seats near the front of the plane to make the whole transition easier. This sounds like a foolproof strategy. No such thing exists in these days of traveling on packed flights where passengers have nothing more than revenue unit status to the airlines.

Another story to demonstrate the inflexibility of airlines.

I had to make a connection for a particular flight. And, as is my rule, since I was feeling great, I decided to forgo the wheelchair to walk. Walking after a flight is the best thing for me physically. I keep the wheelchair as a contingency plan, only necessary if things go badly. On this particular flight I had what I thought would be a great seat, 7D on the aisle at the bulkhead with extra leg room; the extra room allowed me to keep in contact with my feet during the flight. We were in Denver with a "springtime" temperature of 20 degree F. I gave the senior flight attendants my brightest smile and a warm hello to make sure they remembered me, not only because it's the right thing to do, but because it can prove very useful if my situation changes during the flight. It didn't take long. The cabin was cool, not stuffy as it often is. The flight staff prepared for the elusive on-time departure. We made it out of the gate and taxied as scheduled. What could go wrong? Just as we took off the pilot or some member of the crew hit the air-conditioning, and the huge fan directly above me blasted out what seemed like all of that 20 degree air in the Rocky Mountain region.

In the time it took to take off and reach cruising altitude I transitioned from "on" to definitely beyond "off." Sudden blasts of cold seem to affect me negatively. I felt that it might cause hypothermia. The cold increased my shaking which quickly transformed into tremors that were out of control. Parkinson's took over.

This reaction might seem severe, but many others with Parkinson's have described the same reaction to cold blasts. I struggled to put on a light jacket but realized that the shaking was unbounded. This was becoming one of only a few times since I have had Parkinson's that I felt I was headed toward an out-of-control situation. I managed to wave down the flight attendant, having no problem waving with my rapidly gyrating tremor. She was actually looking up and paying attention to the passengers. She was not avoiding eye contact. This was a good sign.

As she came over the senior flight attendant registered that she was just about to deal with someone not in business class. This action apparently is some form of crime. He moved behind her as I began to shake even more, recognizing that stress and trouble were heading my way. When she arrived, I said, "Excuse me, please I'm really cold, could I have a ..."

The senior attendant rudely interrupted. "New rules. We don't give out blankets anymore!"

The first flight attendant looked at me closely. "Are you going into shock?" She apparently noticed that I had lost all my color and that my legs had started to bounce in synchronicity with my hands.

The senior attendant pulled her back into business class where a third flight attendant joined the discussion.

I continued to shake, concerned by the very real possibility that I might lose any degree of control, ultimately earning myself an entry on the no-fly list. At least that was the vision I began to see through my increasing panic. I heard something to the effect of, "I really don't care what the new rules are!"

The junior flight attendant opened a compartment and pulled out a couple of blankets in plastic bags. The third attendant distracted the now angry senior attendant as he tried to reach for the blankets. The first woman was quick and made it down the aisle while the third flight attendant blocked the senior attendant with a very nice basketball pick.

The original attendant wrapped me in blankets and said, "Don't worry we're okay with this."

Whereupon, I stopped thinking about ADA filing status and airline liability issues regarding passenger illness and negligence.

Thinking about my legal standing is a defense mechanism I use to help put a particularly troubling situation in context. This provides an emotionally safe haven and allows me to think about a possible resolution for whatever the current dilemma may be.

In this case the blankets enabled me to hide from the

cold air blast and slowly regain control over my tremors, giving me time to seriously think about my reaction to the psychological feeling of loss of control.

In the early stages Parkinson's sudden presentation of symptoms, symptoms that are not permanent but are harbingers of the future, are very unnerving, even frightening. Sometimes these symptoms are compounded by the side effects of medication. Because I was so stressed and forced to rely on the flight attendant when things went badly, I began to have catastrophic thoughts that nearly pushed me to the point of hallucination. As I have stated before, hallucinations are a side effect of some drugs used in Parkinson's. These are not fleeting problems. They can be serious.

Having flown well over the million mile marker, I have, unfortunately, witnessed passengers die on planes. One of them lay in the aisle next to me halfway to Maui. That was a sobering experience. On a flight to Hong Kong I witnessed three courageous flight attendants work for hours with very unhappy doctors to save the life of a man who seemed to have a stroke. They earned my respect and admiration for their successful efforts.

The dispute among the flight attendant staff left me very anxious and concerned about whether my problem would eventually work itself out. The downside of so much authority being handed to staff who have not trained as EMTs meant the level of motivation and sense of professionalism were highly variable. I was currently working with a house divided and knew that I was soon to be more trouble.

Unfortunately, I knew my next request would ramp up the problem. I would need to use the bathroom and because it was closer to my seat, my only option would be to use the bathroom in business class. This request was complicated because the new security regulations, mixed with the often elite treatment of those in business and first class, prevented a passenger in coach from using the facilities outside their seating area.

The New World says if you're in row seven in economy you must use the bathroom across from row 39 in the back of the plane. If I'm "off," this trek simply is not an option. Tremors and stress seem to accelerate the rate at which my body fills my bladder.

There is a general attitude amongst those flying business class that a business class passenger is entitled to protection from coach travelers. The flight attendants, usually of significant seniority, manage that game very well indeed. The FAA rules on congregating around the pilots' door may be both practical and wise, but my bladder is unconvinced that the potential terror threat changes its actual capacity. Additionally, I am barely able to walk in the cramped quarters of a plane. The aisle is inevitably full of passengers and all the things they stick in the aisle, from elbows to heads to feet. These are obstacles that flight attendants can overcome with the service cart. But to the average passenger, I am just a person who seems to be stumbling his way to the bathroom. This situation can lead to serious conflicts with people who are stressed, exhausted and uncomfortable. How often do we hear about physical confrontations among passengers while airborne?

Once I'd warmed up on this particularly flight, my shaking abated somewhat, and as predicted, I had use the restroom ... soon. I waved the flight attendant back and said, "I'm afraid I'm going to be more trouble."

"Let me guess, you need to use the bathroom in business class," she said.

I nodded, cringing. "I just can't make it 32 rows back."

"Let's go before he sees you coming," she whispered.

I stood up grasping the edge of the bulkhead.

Recognizing that I was likely going to flail in three dimensions and move very slowly she said, "Grab my shoulders."

I did and we began to march forward.

My hands were "tremoring" so they kept squeezing her shoulders on their own. In a desperate attempt to not seem like a weirdo, I cautiously joked "Hope you don't mind the massage."

"No, I need it," she whispered.

The, by-the-rule-book, senior flight attendant stood ahead of us arms crossed and looking perturbed. The third flight attendant ran interference again and pushed the cart into his side. "I need two cabs for 3A and B and another scotch for 5C." He lost his focus and moved out of the way.

I made it into the bathroom and managed to survive by placing my head on the ceiling for balance. When I came out, the third flight attendant was waiting for me with a smile that said, "I'm enjoying this."

"My turn for a massage?" she asked.

"My pleasure." We stepped around the senior flight attendant and moved past passengers who smiled at me and did not show a hint of being affected by the situation.

The irony was that by the time we landed and the plane taxied to the terminal, my body, now very warm and comfortable, had returned to "on." I got up, retrieved my bag from the overhead compartment and woke my wife. With my cane in hand I walked out of the airplane. As I left the plane, I profusely thanked the two flight attendants who had ministered to me and exchanged stares with the senior flight attendant. He looked down at my feet in total disbelief. The female attendants thanked me for their massages as senior attendant spun around looking for something else to do. I don't think all the flight attendants bonded on this leg of the trip.

The attendant who had run interference for the first quietly told me that her father had Parkinson's. In my mind I thanked her father for obviously giving her the sensitivity to understand my problem and disobey the rules formulated by the airline, rules that do not anticipate the needs of disabled passengers. Although this particular experience turned out well for me, it is a lesson about the vulnerability of those with Parkinson's and other disabled individuals in the artificial environment created by modern aircraft. Small changes in the artificial internal environment can be potentially dangerous or harmful obstacles to those whose physiological and psychological states can be destabilized.

There is a clear conflict between the interests of the airline and the needs of disabled passengers, passengers whose limitations are exacerbated and intensified in such a restricted environment. It is reasonable to expect that flight attendants may well see situations differently and ultimately defer to a senior authority. What if the third flight attendant had been rule-driven in this situation? In this era of heightened security, allowing a passenger to use the bathroom in business class, unfortunately located next to the cockpit, might pose a threat to security of the other passengers. However, in retrospect even the senior flight attendant should have acknowledged that that the safety of a passenger outweighed enforcing the blanket rule.

For a person to successfully fly with Parkinson's, the plan for handling such contingencies must be well thought out. Communication with the flight crew and planning ahead may prevent undue stress. Planning ahead and recognizing limitations and triggers will at least help a person to comfortably "go up, up and away."

SECTION 5: EXERCISE
Intervening on Your Own Behalf or Not So Lonely After All

At the time of my Parkinson's diagnosis, I was engaged in a number of sports to stay sane and to try to maintain my health. Although I played handball, skied, golfed, dry fly fished and biked through the mountains of Montana, I had reached a point where most 50-year-old males' bodies have completely adapted to repetitive exercise. My body decided to put on five pounds per year. I believed I was a 6-foot 2-inch, 212-pound athletic male, when in fact I was a 6-foot 1-inch (yes we shrink) 252-pound delusional has-been athlete. As in most cases with males at 54, the phrase, "the older I get the better I was" seemed to fit better than "my best days are ahead."

I had played handball fairly vigorously once or twice a month in my 20s and into my 30s. Since then, while spending my time building a career here in the US and in Asia, I played handball once every six months. Even that implies a regularity that wouldn't be confirmed by a calendar.

For the uninitiated handball is an ancient legendary sport played in the same court as racquetball using a small hard ball which is hit with either hand covered with a light leather glove. Handball is played as singles or doubles, and it is notoriously painful on the hands until the player either becomes skilled or is an old man who feels no pain, at least that he admits to. The great virtue of the sport is a dependence on strategy as well as the added benefit of developing left- and right-side hand-eye coordination and improving agility. In general those who play this sport play with absolute dedication and have designated it, "the perfect sport." The sport is old. In fact the sport may be Egyptian, Irish or Mesoamerican dating to 2000 B.C.

When discussing my diagnosis with a very dear old friend, a stalwart of handball, he suggested that I take the sport up again seriously to see if playing would help me maintain my balance, agility and conditioning. I was mainly impressed that he thought was in good condition and actually had balance and agility. Despite the false premise, I decided he was right, and I could easily return to handball. Of course in my mind I was still somewhere in my 20s and 30s.

Upon my return to the sport, I learned that handball was not just exercise or a fun game that might help me manage my Parkinson's balance and agility issues, but a whole new world, a world made up almost exclusively of older guys, plus a few young people.

It is difficult to describe the relationship between handball players. They play a sport in which participants learn to care for one another through a great deal of healthy competition.

This is sometimes incomprehensible to the outside world.

Chapter 8
Whiskey Friday

"Asshole."

Whew, that must have been a great shot. In fact, that was as high a compliment as I could get around the courts.

"Thanks," I barked, as I flipped him the bird with a big smile, while hitting the next serve off as many walls as I possibly could. He hit a rollout back to me, taking the serve back. As I handed him the ball, under my breath I growled, "Jerk."

"Thanks," he said and promptly served a hard spinning, left hopping ace off the back wall to win the match.

"Nice spitball," I snarled.

"Open your eyes when you swing," he growled.

The other two guys in the room smiled; it was clear that we were old friends. The gruff talk was simply one old dog barking at another from behind a big fence.

Amidst this chaos I reflected briefly on this group of players. Here I was playing handball with an engineer who was 80 years old with two knee replacements; another old jokester who'd had a hip replacement and was fighting cancer; and a 67-year-old, retired airline manager with a pacemaker and a really annoying left fist shot. I was a retired professor with Parkinson's disease and had the mobility of a man with a foot nailed to the floor.

No one can claim, "I'm injured," to explain poor play. Each realizes that we don't have to go far to find ourselves in the company of others who are struggling against some out of control ailments caused by age, disease, or chronic condition. It keeps us humble. We all still seem to think we're playing for the world championship. No one from outside our group would think we could play a sport more physically challenging than Texas hold-um or gin rummy.

In the next court we heard two guys rehashing the previous point. The loser, who thumbed the ball into the floor on the potentially winning point, described himself as a moron, while the winner said, "Yeah, great shot," in a sarcastic voice. This interaction was followed by both men laughing uproariously and agreeing that it was time for whiskey.

As we all hobbled, stumbled and pushed our way out into the hallway from seven different courts, the invasion of smell and noise startled a female racquetball player skipping down the corridor. She flushed, tripped and adjusted her top all in one nanosecond of self-consciousness.

There was a guttural roar in the hallway. On close inspection it was clear the woman had reason to be unsettled. She had just found herself in a closed space with 17 sweaty, smelly men who looked like junkyard dogs.

These men were of every conceivable size, shape, and age. They were dressed in ratty, torn and amazingly discordant clothing stretched over and hung onto their dripping, hairy, yet strangely athletic bodies. At one extreme were five or six men who were 5-feet six-inch to 5-feet 11-inch athletes with zero body fat. At the other end of the spectrum, five or six portly men from 55 to 80 were hobbling, wobbling or limping. Interspersed among these two disparate groups were guys learning the game. They hung back, listening for clues from guys who have played the game for 20 to 60 years and understand the "perfect game." These novices had yet to learn that the longer they played the game the more they would understand the phrase "the longer I play the better I was" as a philosophy, just like it was in the minds of their elders. The stories that emerged during the sipping of the whiskey made that clear.

I recalled a moment in the locker room a few weeks before. One young man aged 30 or so, after being invited to play handball and give up "sissy" racquetball, observed that he was going to wait until he was 50. To him handball seemed to be a painful sport, particularly to the hands. He reasoned that beyond 50, men seemed to feel no pain, so that would be a good time to start.

The group of us who listened to him really had no response to that assessment. Instead, we continued groaning to the music of braces being unbuckled, elbow and knee pads being removed and thoroughly soaked clothing splattering on the floor.

He had smiled confidently and exited with an athletic jump over the bench we were barely able to step over without tripping.

My mind snapped back to the crowded smelly hallway. The moving mass of humanity emerged into an open area where one bottle of Tyrconnell Irish whiskey sat on the table next to the glass walled court we call the "The Cathedral." All were eager for Whiskey Friday to begin. Some raspy voice yelped from the back, "Out of my way, let the lying begin!"

Chapter 9
I Always Wanted to Do That

I wobbled into the locker room and flopped myself down at the end of the bench, exhausted. How much longer would I be able to keep this pace? And, simultaneously, how long I could sustain myself physically without continuing to play. Having just completed three games of handball, decided by no more than four points total in the past two hours, I was whipped. Thank God my medicine held out. As usual both my hands shook, and I wanted to shower and leave before I stiffened up or froze.

From experience, I knew the faster I was, the easier it was to get home and let my meds start their next phase. If I was slowed down by the shakes and still took my meds, I had to stay at the club and wait for them to take effect before I left.

My mind a world of "what ifs," I grabbed my lock and tried to get the combination dialed in. The lock shook and rattled in my left hand, banging against the locker uncontrollably.

After finally selecting the correct number I began to spin the dial other way.

Suddenly a hand appeared over my shoulder and

pinched the knob on the dial spinning the dial in the opposite direction. "I always wanted to do that," said the laughing voice of the guy next to me. Other voices chimed in with light laughter, but with a bit of nervousness.

As I turned to my would-be "buddy," my mind raced. "What to say?" At this moment something very important was being decided within the group. How should I respond to his possible insult?

I knew my decision would affect the tone of our relationship as well as my relationship with the rest of the crowd substantially. My response was, "Jerk, now I'm going to have a hell of time remembering the combination after I kick your ass!"

The crowd roared and my "buddy" knew that the burden of figuring out what to do had been transferred to him.

He processed my response. I'd used the term jerk, a name we handball players call ourselves when we screw up. It was also a term of endearment among those who knew our limitations; we're old, broken down has-beens still trying to play a tough game. My response suggested that my brain may be failing, a common thread of conversation among all of us struggling with being 60 or more. "Kick your ass" was simply a threat that had such hyperbole for someone in my condition it could have no meaning whatsoever.

His response was, "I just couldn't take it anymore, watching and listening to you fumble with that lock every single day. It brings out the devil in me."

This was greeted by some hooting and a few guffaws.

"So that's all it takes?" someone in the background asked.

"If I had known that I would've gotten a bigger, louder lock," I said.

There was considerable laughter to this response.

"You know I'd buy one for you. I'm generous!" my friend retorted.

After this exchange, the locker room returned to the ongoing deception of pretending we were athletes in our prime simply recovering from a strenuous workout. Everyone attempted to shed the look of junkyard dogs and transform into something sort of presentable in order to return to civilization. My friend and I shook hands and had a belly laugh. We had cemented a friendship that we trusted could last for years.

As time as gone by, we both still laugh as I fumble with my lock, and he shakes his head remembering his off the wall action. This helps me calm down and get into my locker quietly. Occasionally, I still feel a devilish urge to bang the lock on the locker just to be annoying.

People who interact with someone with Parkinson's have varied reactions. Some people use dark humor, while others just don't know how to respond. Those of us with Parkinson's have the opportunity to use humor and language to help them deal with the problem.

People with PD have symptoms which to others might seem a variety of weirdly expressed actions: shaking, twisting, turning and freezing in place. These manifestations of the disease make one unable to move and cause us to do things like bang one's lock on the locker. A person with PD must be prepared for those around him to struggle to treat these symptoms as normal behavior.

Someone with Parkinson's is like a random number cue generator. PD complicates situations that others take for granted. It is no surprise if someone with PD disturbs a normal situation, people will react in unanticipated ways. I have found that since I've had PD that I have some success with others if I anticipate and accommodate their reaction to me. I take a wait-and-see attitude and size up the situation from their point of view as best I can.

Chapter 10
"Could You Dry This Off for Us?"

Some years ago an old hand at the game began joining our handball games. I had never met him before he joined us; he was an interesting character likely to be found in a place like Butte, Montana; Clarion, Pennsylvania or any rough industrial town in America. He was a bowlegged tough Irishman with a quick sense of humor. We immediately got along. But as we played handball I could see he was somewhat uncomfortable when my Parkinson's symptoms appeared during games. We always played doubles, but he was never my partner.

One particular day the game was close and fairly intense. At one point the ball hit my very sweaty partner and bounced into the Irishman's hands. He looked down at the dripping ball and up at me with my shaking hands. I was ready to serve. He hesitated. Then he sort of smiled and rather than throw me the ball he stepped forward a couple of steps and held it out. "Could you dry this off for us?" he asked.

"Okay," I replied, "but hold it out at arms-length so the wind does not mess up your hair."

Everybody laughed. He wiped the ball on his shorts, rubbed it in his gloves, flipped it to me and said, "Play on guys."

After that experience, we played as partners for years.

He had resolved his discomfort with my Parkinson's symptoms by directly confronting the symptom itself. Actually what he was addressing was my perception of how others viewed my symptoms. Did he feel he had to give me some slack or not?

Slack is a confusing word and a negatively loaded concept in this context. No one wants to ask for "some slack." But the reality is that adjustments may need to be made. There is often uncertainty of how to make the adjustments with good grace at the time they occur so the game can continue. To avoid confusion this issue needs to be dealt with openly, directly and immediately, as my friend did. With a little humor, and the ability to recognize and communicate each person's uncertainty regarding the limitations of the other, it is possible to overcome some of these social obstacles without permanently altering the nature of the game.

When Parkinson's invades one's life, even a reasonably well-adjusted person will experience a transformation that inevitably tends to make him or her self-centered. Individuals with PD are constantly monitoring themselves and must learn to deal with their changing motor functions and capacities. At the most extreme end of the spectrum, the self-centered behavior can be demanding, controlling and certainly off-putting to those they come in contact with.

As individuals develop ways to compensate for the negative effects of Parkinson's, it is important they keep a watchful eye on not becoming self-centered in social situations. Those with PD often focus their mind on their symptoms in settings where they are very active. These situations tend to be events where people with PD feel vulnerable both physically and socially. A self-absorbed focus yields a kind of self-conscious if not selfish demeanor. My experience has been 99 percent positive if I approach the situation by allowing vulnerabilities to show, at least to some degree. This allows others to make adjustments and determine how to address the situation without being intrusive or standoffish.

Locker rooms have always been places where people, at least in my experience, let their guard down. They commiserate and replay moments and through conversation and humor, diffuse competition, both on and off the court. The type of activity, be it handball, tennis, weightlifting or yoga, determines the styles of behavior. If an individual with PD is still able maintain this sustained level of physical activity with Parkinson's, they are fortunate. The need to pay close attention to their physical health means that individuals with PD need to participate more in these active, social situations. Recent studies on exercise and intense exercise, such as riding a bicycle at 90 RPMs for an hour, seem to show that Parkinson's symptoms can be alleviated for a while by intense physical exercise. The body produces more dopamine during heightened states of activity. No matter how people with PD manage exercise, they are going to be in the company of committed athletes.

The fact that our handball group included people with knee and hip replacements, shoulder and back surgeries and pacemakers, as well as cancer survivors among other ailments meant everyone just played on. No one used their impairment as an excuse for missing a shot, let alone losing a game.

To illustrate this point, one of the members of the handball group, a former champion at the local and national level, has Meniere's disease. During matches he will have what appears to be a seizure (It is actually an attack of vertigo.), and he will collapse to the floor, sometimes incapacitated for about 15 minutes. When this occurs, his doubles partners make sure he is comfortable on the floor and talk until he recovers. Play then resumes with no penalties. The bigger issue is remembering the score as well as explaining to outsiders why there is a guy lying on court floor. It's amazing how often people respond with a simple, "Okay," as if this situation was perfectly normal.

The humor and seemingly ornery behavior within our handball group has allowed us to test our limitations, challenge our preconceived notions on both sides and find common ground. The other members don't have to worry about limiting their fun because of my symptoms, and I don't have to worry about hiding my symptoms to pretend to still be normal. The question most often asked by people dealing with physical disabilities is, "Do I treat PD as a disqualifier and stop playing, or do I forget about it and just play the game despite some limitations?" I can assure you in the vast majority of the cases people just want to play the game. They are happy to have someone with whom to play despite their opponent's limitations. Sometimes limitations are assets when tested in a real situation rather than prejudged with no opportunity to explore the real effect of an apparent shortcoming.

The game of baseball begins when the umpire says, "Play ball." The umpire never starts a game by saying, "Be sensitive." Individuals who have Parkinson's are well served by making sure that the game goes on and to do their best to have fun participating at whatever level they can.

Chapter 11
"Okay, Everybody, Let's Call It a Mulligan"

Golf is a peculiar game. It uses a range of skills, from gross motor skills down to precise hand-eye coordination skills in an outdoor environment with a pace of activity that ranges from almost sleeping to the excitement of a home run in baseball. Yes, I've seen a golfer fall asleep and fall out of a golf cart. Although, I must admit, I'm not sure what was in his water bottle.

Golf is sometimes played by those who engage only with a fixed foursome, a kind of locked-in social group. Due to the complexity of scheduling, it is common for an individual faced with cancellation by a friend, to join a twosome arranged by the golf course. The third alternative is either wandering out alone or being placed on a team raising money for a crusade, such as a Parkinson's fundraiser. In the third case you're on your own.

I played about five years of golf before my Parkinson's journey began. My one skill was hitting the ball very far, likely due to learning to throw things in high school, such as the shot put and discus. As these activities required throwing an object far with little control of where it goes, this method could explain my golf shot. Great distance was achieved but with directional impairment.

A friend of mine and I managed to find a lovely golf course to play in the Flathead Valley in Montana. The views are unmatched. The course layout had the number one tee box right next to the ninth green which meant the two fairways converged like a V for victory roughly at the tee box on the first hole. The starter's shack was set up facing the first tee box.

In Montana some people have personal spaces that cover acres, and their view of property rights tends toward "my property is absolutely mine and yours sort of is also." Since all the golfers shared this philosophy, hitting into the group on the nearby hole a couple of times could lead to conflict. As a result, the wise managers of the course had assigned an employee to be the starter on hole number one. It was the employee's task to separate the foursomes by eight minutes to keep potential riots on the fifth hole to a minimum.

On this particular day, my friend and I were paired with two other guys who definitely were cocky, but old, and had not quite yet come to terms with the idea that their best days were behind them. We thought this was normal. Our companions were soon staring at us. I, of course, was shaking like a leaf, my hands moving like I was trying to keep time with Charlie Parker at his bebop best. My friend ignored my shaking completely. He commenced hitting practice shots with his 7-iron, digging up clumps of grass that were the size of the sod used to replace a lawn. We carefully replaced the divots, pouring a little water around each one.

The two hot guys took their turn on the tee box and nicely hit drives 220 yards down the center of the fairway. My friend took his 7-iron and wildly hit the big ball first, a golf term for burying the club in the ground, sending clumps of Earth 60 yards in a spraying arc. His drive managed to land 50 yards into the rough. I sensed his frustration and offered him some encouragement. "Nice drive."

"Yeah, thanks," he responded. "Is the ground this hard everywhere?"

On the way to the white markers, I froze up a couple times, and my hands shook enough that it took three stabs of the tee to place my ball on the ground. I had to reset the ball twice before I was ready.

My driver was black and yellow, about the size of a bowling ball cut in half. The name Sasquatch was prominently displayed on the backside. Just between shakes I began my swing, yielding a drive about 270 yards down the ninth fairway. This caused a huge number of people to scramble. Knowing my first drives are usually wild to the left, I yelled, "fore."

Immediately the starter leapt out of the starting shack to count the dead. It was a line drive.

"That usually happens on my first drive when the driving range is closed," I explained. I also shouted, "I can correct it!" and sort of bowed an apology to the crowd to my left and behind me.

"Okay, but let's call it a Mulligan," he said. "I will get the ball. Everybody behind the starter shack, now!"

This was great because as I looked down the first fairway, even in my peripheral vision, I had no audience. I was able to relax and easily convert my fine muscle shaking into gross motor movement and, with a nice easy swing, hit a drive about 230 yards down the fairway.

Suddenly we discovered that we were a twosome. The starter just said, "Keep going, but I want to hear you yell 'fore' frequently." We agreed and played our typical game, seeing a lot of the course with intermittent conversation. We also had the bonus of two nice Pro V1 Titleist golf balls waiting for us about 220 yards down the fairway.

I never got to explain to the competitive pair that I have Parkinson's, and I still can play golf, once I am warmed up.

My friend offered a consolation. "Hey, this situation is

better than the last time. Remember the guys who wanted to place some bets on the score, and we explained that you had Parkinson's and didn't bet on golf? They said it was no fun to play if there wasn't something on the line, so we went ahead and played for lunch money and beers over the first nine holes, winner buys. Remember how quiet the lunch was?"

All I remembered was that I kept trying to explain to them that I wasn't a shill, and I had no idea how shaking didn't interfere with my golf game. I still feel it has something to do with switching concentration from the section of my brain that manages tremors and walking to the section that focuses on golf. I do not think they bought the story. However, by the end of 18 holes their understanding had been completely reversed. So had the score, and as a result, the beer was on us.

This type of situation occurs frequently with Parkinson's since, try as I might, it is very difficult to get people to understand the strangeness of Parkinson's. Its physical manifestations are often abstract. The most difficult characteristic occurs when I am unable to walk, frozen in place, then appear normal 10 minutes later. My friend has listened to me over the years and observed this unpredictable phenomenon, matching my patience with his own. As a result my erratic behavior is normal to him. Not everyone will walk down the road with an unpredictable person armed with golf clubs.

When someone places a limit on their tolerance of issues faced by the disabled, it stunts their ability to learn from the breadth of human experience. But that is their problem. An individual with Parkinson's has the choice to either ignore someone who is limited or attempt to expand their point of reference. However, I=isolation in the face of rejection is not acceptable. Despite the social difficulties that might arise due to others' perception of Parkinson's, it is crucial to show up.

Because it takes a long time to play the game, I have

found golf to be an especially good environment to work on educating people about Parkinson's. Nine holes can take two and a half hours, assuming there are no fights on the fifth hole. Eighteen holes can take four hours or more, assuming there is no major lunch break after nine holes. It is easy to learn a great deal about other people, and it is very difficult to hide the symptoms of Parkinson's in that amount of time. In four and half hours I normally go through a complete cycle of medicine and a full complement of symptoms ranging from normal to shaking, then a stumbling walk back to normal. If we'd had the opportunity to convince those two competitive golfers to continue playing, I think it would've gone very differently; perhaps more like an experience I had at a wedding golf tourney.

In the wedding tournament we were grouped into foursomes. The groups were set up as two men, two women, with a skilled man and a skilled woman on each team paired with two weaker players. I was the weak male, obviously. As we began, the skilled male player, who had conquered significant health problems, seemed somewhat listless and was not hitting the ball well. He assigned the blame to general soreness. He also seemed slightly irritated with my disruptive activities. I was busy making the other tourney players nervous with my directionally impaired shots flying around the course. Our skilled woman partner was very consistent, and we were posting a fairly good string of pars as a foursome.

My struggles were close to forcing me to quit because I could hardly get up on the tee boxes. I was almost unable to get across the greens to putt without shuffling my feet; with the golf cleats this could damage the greens. At some point, I sensed that the skilled golfer began to watch my struggle and pay less attention to his as we moved through the first five holes.

On the sixth hole I barely made it to the tee box from the cart. Unbeknownst to anyone within my party, my medicine was improving my tremor but not my gait. This was a 175-yard par three hole. I hit the ball to within three feet of the pin. As I often say, "golf broke out." A quick putt, and we had a birdie and were one below par after six.

With some more marvelous shots by the skilled woman we started to join the competition. The skilled guy asked me how I was able to adjust so quickly, thus losing any focus on his own discomfort and pain. I had two or three shots that kept us under par, and it was clear to him that the medicine was working. Soon we were pulling together as a team, a crucial aspect of this experience.

This change in perspective for the skilled male golfer improved his attitude. That, combined with the skilled woman's consistency and clever sense of the game kept our score at or below par through the middle holes. However, by the 16th hole my tremor returned, and I began to stiffen up which made walking more difficult. Our fourth, a nurse, recognized immediately that due to the heat and thus likely dehydration, I had cycled through my medication very quickly. Her diagnosis was correct, and she literally kept me afloat with her thoughtfulness and water bottles.

I sensed that the skilled golfer had something to say to me. At one point we passed each other, and he apologized, "Sorry about the first few holes. I had my head in the wrong place." We looked at each other and laughed at all the potential meanings. "It matters that you don't give in to being self-absorbed doesn't it?" he continued.

"Today went well, thanks. How's the pain? A beer might help," I replied.

He smiled and shrugged. "The pain? We're under par for 17. What pain? You're up."

We were on the 18th hole with a 40 foot gnarly putt, and I was up. Between tremors I managed to get it within a foot or so. He dropped it in the hole, and we finished one under par. With a few high-fives as we walked off the course we knew we had made a great day out of one that could've gotten away from us. I could've easily quit. He could've easily spoiled his day, and the combination would've ruined the experience for the two stalwart women we played with. Not only is showing up crucial. We depend on each other, so an opportunity to learn how others cope is an experience that benefits all.

SECTION 6: CHILDREN
Being Charmed

Children can be cautious, insightful and curious all at the same time. When confronted with an adult who otherwise looks normal but who might shake or freeze in place and sometimes has trouble negotiating corners, children often act as though they discovered some stranger who needs to be announced to the world or as a new species of human. Frequently their reaction is conveyed with a frankness that makes one smile at their pure innocence. Their words aren't carefully chosen, couched in offensive stereotypes or dressed up in current political correctness. They just state what they see.

When I encounter children, generally between the ages of eight and two, their reactions prompt me to inwardly chuckle, but still be very cautious, especially when I am "off." We all have the experience of knowing we're being stared at; few stares are more penetrating than those of a child. I try to meet them met with a smile that's friendly.

Sometimes children will simply approach and want to play. They inevitably ask a cosmic level question such as, "Why can't you walk?" When the walking stick is tapping the floor, they will ask to use it for some tapping of their own. Other children will get near enough to catch my attention and then retreat to their parents or babysitter, all the while indicating they want to stay and find out what's going on with me.

One surprising aspect is their tendency to instinctively want to help despite the confusion associated with dealing with an adult who is not completely in control. They are usually not used to that situation unless they have grandparents. As they ponder what to do to help an adult, their behavior often foreshadows the potential adult they will transition into. This is a great teaching moment to help them investigate the effect of their own approach to the world around them. It can be fun.

Experiences of this sort are an inevitable occurrence in the day-to-day life for someone with Parkinson's. Traveling, shopping, going out to eat and taking a walk have led to many encounters with children that are very memorable. The next section describes two encounters with children that have made a lasting impression on me.

Chapter 12
"Hey Mom, That Man over There Can Read a Book While It's Moving"

Flying a commercial airplane is one of the most offensively public yet painfully private experiences we endure. Flying in economy always raises the specter of those who are in favor of deregulation. I once observed a 6-foot 5-inch, 280-pound weightlifter unable to get to his peanuts because he couldn't open the package. I couldn't help being amused as I watched him struggle with the package biting it, tearing at it, pounding it on the armrest. This was a great depiction of the inconvenience and discomfort of airline travel. It reminded me that the general problem with society is making people think that they might die not from terrorism, but from packaging.

The real terrorists have won the battle because by causing an infinitely small probability that there be might be an attack, they've made a certainty out of the fact that travelers will be angry at their seat, the attendant, fellow passengers, the airline, the FAA, the Congress and the President. The terrorists are fomenting revolution one peanut package at a time. It's the little things that really bog us down and force us to say "enough."

For me, the only realistic escape from travel problems is to either fall dead asleep in a coma-like state or to read. Since I shake, and because I worry that if I do fall asleep on the plane my legs will never, ever work again, I read. This means that I need to have a light on, something to hold my head up, something to rest the book on and my reading glasses. Getting all this organized keeps me active and attracts attention. Mixed in with the frustrated and stressed adults are confused children who begin to act out their reaction to the confinement being imposed on them. We all recognize the signs: kicking the backs of seats, pounding the keys on noisy toys and random loud and continuous commentary, only broken up by the familiar phrases of "When do we get there?" or "Bobby hit me first." One of these distractions is repeated every time I relax and begin a new chapter and is often followed by "Use your inside voice, honey."

While all this is happening, other things are going on as well. The attendant, without being asked, brings water and asks that I let her know if this water is enough for my medication. The huge guy in front of me twists back as he sits down and asks if it is okay to put the seat back halfway. The parent behind me requests that you let them know if the kid's games are too loud or obnoxious. The person the aisle across tells me they've got my back if I need help to the bathroom. The college student in the window seat leans over and asks if I am interested in eating the rest of their Vietnamese satay and pot stickers.

Others hear the civilized approaches, and a wave of courtesy flows back down the aisle. Civil society in fact emerges one little detail at a time. Our subconscious musings often paint a scene that is either/or, creating a revolution or a civil society. Most of the time my experience is that reality is going to be neither our worst nightmare nor our most delightful dream.

After things settled down, I began reading my latest 1000-page book; this one by Ken Follett about 11th-century cathedrals in England and Europe.

I was somewhere between sleep and reading when I heard, "Hey Mom, that guy up there can read a book while it's moving!" This was delivered in a stage whisper that no one around me could miss. This sort of woke me up, and I looked around, catching the guy across the aisle from me smiling, and the mother across the aisle behind me blushing and looking squeamish. The kid did not blink.

I didn't really know what to do, so I smiled and motioned him to talk with me. As I did, the person sitting in the middle seat next to me whispered, "He was standing in the aisle the last 12 minutes or so utterly mesmerized." The guy across the aisle said, "How do you do that?" Unbeknownst to me, I had become sort of a strange curiosity to those who could see my hands shaking this 1000-page book while calmly reading and turning the pages for the last hour or so. The book was so huge and thick I often considered it a personal defense weapon as well as a fine read, but it did require me to wedge it in between the fold-down tray and my belt in order to keep it from shaking too wildly.

The kid came forward. "Yeah, how do you do that?"

I smiled. "I really didn't realize I was reading a moving book. You see, for me, the book and my eyes move together so the only thing that I see moving is the plane."

At that point the kid stared at me. This made me realize that he was either worried about my shaking or my sanity because I am sure he was fairly clear in his mind the plane was not shaking. It was the book.

"I have Parkinson's disease, and it makes my hands shake," I said. "I can't make them stop, so in order to read I must have learned to train my eyes to move with the book. I didn't even know I was doing it."

"It's like when you're riding a horse," the kid replied.

"You just move your legs and your hands, and the horse does what you want."

It was clear I was on a plane leaving Montana.

"Yeah that's right," I responded, "and you don't even have to think about it."

The kid smiled.

"Now don't bother the man anymore," the mother interrupted.

"He's not bothering me," I explained. "He's educating me."

The kid headed to his seat, satisfied that he'd worked this puzzle out in his head.

As I turned back to my book, the guy across the aisle smiled and said "smart kid."

"I sure never had a horse like that," the guy next to me stated.

"Now that I know what's going on with my reading I wonder if I'll be able to do it anymore?" I commented to them both.

We all three laughed, and, in chorus, they both wished me good luck. "Here goes nothing." I said. Within five minutes or so I was oblivious to the book movement, but I noticed when I looked up there was one little blue eye peering at the book between the seats in front of me watching the motion.

Another child had fixated on my movements.

Chapter 13
Little Man, Little Boy

Grandchildren are amazing in that they represent an unusual reality. In my mind they are a chance to perfect the work and concepts employed in rearing one of their parents, but in reality they are different, the times are different and you are different. I also believed grandchildren are proof of the magical theory that it would be easier for fathers if they could have a second child first so that they could begin rearing children as an experienced parent. Slipping into this line of logic seemed wholly realistic for me as a grandparent. It was a bit of a delusion, of course. The reality is much different. My grandchildren are, in fact, my children's creation. Grandchildren instinctively see grandparents as secondary sources for their primary needs. It is easy for a grandparent to confuse their own needs with reality.

My Parkinson's diagnosis concerned me as a grandparent. I worried that my grandchildren would only remember me as someone who shakes, freezes in place and is sometimes stuck in a chair. Because I have very little endurance I can't participate in many activities for long. In fact, like it or not, my grandchildren will remember me like this because there is no denying my symptoms are the reality.

My daughter is not only a parent now, but also sometimes parents me. She recently reassured me by stating simply, "Children are narrowly focused. If you're lying on the floor having spasms, but you are playing with them, they will remember the play, not the fact that you were gyrating like a fish out of water."

One of the great joys of having grandchildren close by is the pleasure of spontaneously having dinner together. On one special occasion, after an afternoon of playing games invented by my grandchildren involving variations of basketball, foursquare, dodge ball and watching me do something crazy on the jungle gym, I became exhausted. I began to shake and get rigid. This state is a sure signal to go inside, take my medicine and sit down for a while. Sometimes when I take a break my symptoms abate, sometimes they do not. In fact they may even get worse.

Unfortunately, a break did not help. The four grandchildren came in, continuing the exciting act of charging about laughing, screeching and having a great time. When it was time to go to dinner, I found myself 40 feet away from the table standing on polished hardwood floors frozen in place. As I tried to organize my body to take a step, it was clear my brain had internalized the slickness of the floor, the natural fear of falling dominated any motor control I might have had. Both of my hands were shaking out of control as well. What now? I desperately didn't want to ask the children for help.

Suddenly a little hand grabbed mine firmly, and a small voice simply said, "I gotcha Den." This cracked apart the Parkinson's freeze, and I took a step forward. The tiny hand supported me, moving forward with just the right assistance. We moved to the dinner table where the chair was properly turned so that I could sit down without having to spin.

"Have you got it?" the little big man voice asked.

"You betcha," I answered.

With that signal my five-year-old grandson reverted to form, yelled "Yippee!" and with cape flying, ran out of the dining room, hit the hall at maximum speed and skidded down the floor in his socks yelling, "Spiderman rules!"

None of the adults paid attention to this exchange with my grandson. I relied on the advice from my daughter: Don't worry, play. Even the youngest of children knows how to be helpful when you need him to be. My beautiful granddaughters have added numerous instances where they have morphed from being a child to being caregivers so seamlessly that time might have stopped, but not the flow of play. I never really have asked for help; they just appear saying something like, "Can I carry your walking stick?" or "Let me take your hand." These experiences remind me of phrases I used to hear in the old Caribbean, "Don't worry, be happy, no dramas."

SECTION 7: INTERVENORS

In this book I make the following observation that good people are helpful sometimes which is a generalization. I think my experience over time suggests that this is true over the course of one's life.

People rise to the occasion when they see someone engaged in a battle with body control. Almost all of us are aware that unpredictable forces are capable of damaging our mobility. We know when we see a person unable to walk, for example, that in a heartbeat what we are observing, we could be experiencing. Those who have this connection to people in a predicament instinctively step in to help. Those who do not help, I believe may eventually step forward in the future, when they make the connection that one day they could have a movement disorder such as Parkinson's.

Never having been remotely disabled prior to being diagnosed with Parkinson's, I didn't pay a great deal of attention to who helped and who did not in circumstances where someone needed assistance. In my household as I grew up the mantra was, "protect and serve." My father was a policeman. This was emblazoned on his uniforms and badges and even on the side of the police cars. It was pretty clear that my father believed in this view of the world. As a result I tended to be a person who helped, and I noticed in numerous circumstances that I was rarely alone.

Now that I am often caught in Parkinson's related predicaments, I am the beneficiary of the helpers who appear of nowhere at the right moment to assist with the situation and then, as quickly as they arrived, vanish into thin air. Sometimes the intervention is unnecessary, and they are uniformly gracious when thanked for the offer. Sometimes the intervention is more than is needed and has to be handled delicately. And in some situations the help is not about apparent needs of the disabled but rather the person's understanding of the situation. This last situation calls on communication skills that need to be clear yet discreet. If there is good communication, the situation can be resolved instead of becoming overwhelming. For people with Parkinson's, the feeling of being "outnumbered" is associated with too many things needing to be done at once. Providing an extra hand or just serving as backup can make the difference between success and failure in solving the problem.

Chapter 14
Hells Angels

After 10 years of living with Parkinson's, a person learns that travel is risky. Traveling requires entering the crazy land of promises like, "handicapped accessible" which often amounts to "already being used" by someone who isn't handicapped. This crazy land includes "traffic areas," which often mean "obstructions abound," obstacles created by architects who have lost sight of practical needs when designing human traffic areas. However, one tends to bravely sally forth because a person needs a change, new scenery. And, very importantly, a caregiver/partner sometimes needs a change even more.

In this particular instance, the trip seemed very sane and well-managed. Not only was the trip designed for seniors engaged in lifelong learning, but I was a member of the organization arranging the trip. Thus, it seemed that everything would be carefully controlled. The trip was an overnight to that magnificent part of Montana where Charlie Russell painted with brilliant, beautiful colors to capture the majesty of the Great Plains and the power of the upper Missouri River. Charlie Russell added cowboys to his work which gave the paintings their special Russell style. The cowboys of the Russell era are long gone from this part of Montana, so we were there to enjoy the landscape and hear tales about the heroic cowboys from frontier days.

On the first day everything went well. Then fatigue set in. For the first time ever, I found myself in need of a wheelchair. I'd learned to negotiate in a wheelchair way back when I was 16 and had a knee injury from football. Having managed the first day's experience on this trip without a wheelchair, I felt very confident. I'd had fantastic help, maybe even more than I needed, to make sure I got around efficiently. Unfortunately, it was the second day that I encountered a real problem.

We had managed to get to the stunning viewing center above the Great Falls of the Missouri River so that we could see the power of the falls that forced Lewis and Clark to portage their heavy boats many miles overland, basically ending their river trip up the Missouri.

I sat in the wheelchair in the back of a magnificent auditorium watching a slide show and narration of the Lewis and Clark expedition. Approximately 80 of us were all settled down in the dark when the doors opened. In walked two completely costumed Hells Angels. They appeared typical of this subculture, one about 6 foot 6 and about 305 pounds, the other a rangy 5 feet 10 inches and 135 pounds. The only thing they had in common with the group was gray hair. The difference was that their gray hair was blown back because they had been roaring across the Great Plains, obviously without helmets.

As they moved across the room, their leather pants rubbed together, and their heavy boots resounded on the floor. They slowly sat down accompanied by big thumps. Everybody in the room registered their entrance and carefully returned attention to the screening of our Montana history. Strangely, the characters depicted in the Lewis and Clark pictographs looked more like the Hells Angels than the modern Montanans in our group. I think this similarity was lost on the crowd.

Then the show ended. The lights came up. I realized that I had barely enough time to make it to the bathroom. I had kept Mother Nature at bay, not wanting to open the doors again, bringing in the flash of light which would have created another distraction for the crowd. Now was the time to move. So I grabbed the wheels, spun them as fast as I could, and rolled into the foyer seeking the men's restroom. My wife and some friends were right behind me, all of whom were heading to the ladies' restroom.

I managed to get through the interior 12-foot tall glass doors and locate the bathroom which, fortunately, had a handicapped sign on it. I breathed a sigh of relief. I wheeled around the corner and realized immediately I was in deep trouble. The deep trouble was that the handicapped component must have referred to a large stall inside the bathroom. This designation ignored the configuration of the door into the restroom. The entry door, both in size and weight, looked like a door that would be considered grizzly bear proof. Ironically, this kind of massive door becomes an insurmountable barrier to the bathroom even though there are accessibility modifications inside the stalls. This type of design flaw is not uncommon. The door was virtually unreachable from a wheelchair, so I pulled up to it sideways and attempted to push the door open trying to edge the wheelchair in slowly. The size and weight of the door made this attempt nearly impossible. But the deciding factor was the overbuilt spring. It was so resistant it pushed my wheelchair slightly sideways and backwards. Despite all my efforts, the door didn't budge. In fact, I lost ground when I pushed against it.

There I sat, sort of dazed by the "what the hell do I do now" thought raging through my brain. I began to believe I might urinate on the floor. All of a sudden, I started to move backwards, spinning slightly. The figure stepping in front of me was the smaller Hells Angel; I'll call him Slim. Slim pushed the door open and with astonishing speed and pinpoint accuracy the larger Hells Angel, (I'll call him Sir) moved me through the entrance carefully without crushing my fingers. Not a word was spoken.

At the far end of the stalls a man who obviously needed a great deal of space started to walk nimbly into the handicapped stall. Sir growled a sort of "uh-uh" sound. The gentleman's eyes opened wide as Slim cut him off. The man suddenly decided his timing was off, and his space needs had been reduced substantially. As the lead man, Slim declared, "All's clear."

I was moved into the stall. I heard a kind of muffled, "We'll wait." A little time passed, and the door opened after I flushed. There they stood. Again, Slim handled the stall door as Sir managed to squeeze around and behind me, giving me the feeling that he was pushing the walls slightly backward as we began the trip to the sink. At that point, I started to say something and Sir mumbled, "It's okay. We got this, friend."

They quickly moved me through the bathroom out the massive door returning me to the foyer. At that point, I finally managed to get the words out. "You guys are great."

"We don't hear that much," Sir said.

Just then some of the ladies emerged from the bathroom to see the Hells Angels pat me on the back and head out the main exit.

As I looked for my wife, I heard the roar of their motorcycles. It reminded me of the ending of every episode of The Lone Ranger, "Hi Ho Silver Away." And it made me think about the fact that although the heroic frontier cowboys were gone from this scene, they were replaced by these two unlikely gentlemen who appeared in this moment. In my mind the name Hells Angels made me harken back to the uncanny resemblance these long haired, bearded, rough men had to the long haired, bearded, tough members of the Lewis and Clark expedition the crowd was just admiring. The crowd did not seem to notice that there was something significant to respect in these two Hells Angels as well. As Slim and Sir left, a distinct tension in the crowd vanished.

Had I just witnessed "Undaunted Courage"? No, just what used to be called "common courtesy." This experience reminded me that the people who step forward to help a person in a predicament are those who, in that moment, connect you to something familiar in their lives, motivating them to help. It is my belief that those who don't step forward in one instance will eventually find a connection and step up to the challenge in the future. Thus, I learned an important lesson from this experience. The assistance a person receives may come from a completely unexpected source. And popular perceptions about the behavior of subgroups in society may be a poor guide to their actual behavior. I'm now a fan of road warriors and the roar of a Harley.

Chapter 15
Intermission

One of the great joys of living in a small university town is the sheer pleasure of having literally hundreds of concerts, lectures, classes, sporting events and fundraisers to choose from in any given year and sometimes any given month. Though we often think that such a cornucopia of choices would create endless diversion, it also creates something akin to the choice among toothpastes in the local store. With literally 120 different varieties of toothpaste, people just stand there in total paralysis trying to figure out which enemy of plaque is needed. The decision is impossible!

In the world of entertainment choice, if a person has Parkinson's, a decision must include adding crowd effects to the complexity of choosing which event to attend. Parkinson's has an insidious quality which produces anxiety. Dealing with anxiety is a complex issue. Until it's resolved, one's mind just keeps moving through possible scenarios rather than what is probable. Focusing on what is probable requires help to stay grounded.

With any disability, part of the decision is the daunting interaction of logistics and dealing with the reality of being in public space. I understand Parkinson's, so the picture of sitting in my seat enjoying the event is counterbalanced by a game consisting of figuring out how many doors will be involved, how far the walk will be, wondering if the floors are flat, whether there are many stairs and the weather at the current moment. Am I likely to face ice, snow, water and puddles, wind or, in the case of Montana, all these at once?

When I work all that out, I have to take into account the way in which the university is set up as a unit and recognize that individual citizens who use the campus will be going from place to place in a great rush. Universities are peculiar free-form movement areas in that they try to organize the whole campus organically so that nothing dies in transit. In contrast the campus citizens organize their own individual behaviors much like a herd of cats trying to get to where they must be at the moment without regard to their own or anyone else's safety. Students behave as though they have nine lives and will always land on their feet. This contest between the whole and the parts is not unique to Montana. Walking in Manhattan around Christmas, walking anywhere in Italy, trying to cross the street in Bangkok, thinking about going to China and understanding why I never want to go back to Calcutta keeps me alert to "traffic" issues.

The difference in the university setting is that the vast majority of the students are between the ages of 18 and 25. In my former life as a university professor, I had attained a certain status where they needed me to survive. Students could miraculously pick professors out of the crowd. Somehow they sensed that we were the key to getting a degree for which they had taken out massive student loans. They needed to protect their investment.

Through my eyes students were for the most part traveling random performance artists on devices that include bicycles, skateboards, Rollerblades, tennis shoes with little rollers on them, motorized scooters, recumbent bikes, unicycles, shopping carts and racing wheelchairs. The extra added attraction these days was that they were all texting and/or on their cell phones at the same time. Even the ones walking moved in tight packs all focused inwardly, with some walking backwards and others dancing around the edges seeking attention.

Given that state, why would a person with Parkinson's ever enter the danger zone of a university campus? The answer comes from my wife and caregiver when she snaps her fingers as I am mentally working my way through the worst scenario.

"I know what you thinking," she says. "I can read it in your eyes. Each of the things you fear has happened maybe once or twice over the last 35 years. All we're doing tonight is going to a little concert that lasts about three hours."

She's right. Even in my agitated state I can do the math; 35 years includes 306,810 hours, and I've witnessed 20 incidents that could potentially be terrifying in those 35 years. That works out to one chance in 5,114 that something is likely to go wrong in the three hours we'd be on campus.

Okay, I'm going out tonight!

Now is the time to get dressed. "I'll dress in layers to deal with any weather pattern, put on knee pads and elbow pads, a flak jacket, a baseball hardhat, the old hockey gloves and my ancient Basque hiking boots," I muse.

"No jeans tonight. We're getting dressed up, so try out your new slacks," my wife comments above the noise of the hairdryer,

My spouse has broken the muse and reality sets in again. So I leave in my nice sweater, slacks and dress shoes. I pick out my wooden cane which in my mind is actually a Makalu walking stick with an ice penetrating spike on the third extension. Reality returns, and with no margin of security against the improbable, off I go to a night of the Komodo Drummers. This event, chosen for social reasons I learned later, is not a perfect fit. Right now getting to the building is the primary focus. As we both near campus, my ever vigilant wife says, "I think you are brave." A little silence follows. I later learn that's not all I need to be.

As I sit in my aisle seat I can't believe I made it without any serious incident. The only issue was a bit of congestion as we entered the theater. I had some involuntary, and yes annoying, tapping of my walking stick on the floor. But everyone very courteously let me sally forth, and I am sitting.

Now the stage is full of half-naked Japanese drummers hammering away at drums from the size of pumpkins to the width of giant tires on trucks that haul iron ore out of the ground of some open pit mine. My heart and my shakes are now all moving in unison to this scene that appears to precede the end of days.

This adjustment is automatic for the shaking and muscle contractions in Parkinson's. I have learned that this bizarre syncopation of body movement and outside noise is par for the course whenever one goes to hear really loud music or even when one is dogged by a mowing machine while playing golf, or when someone is using a grass trimmer or a leaf blower. I have learned to work with it and hold on to the understanding that what's actually happening is not a major cardiac arrest.

A certain kind of uneasiness begins to emerge in the audience which tells me that intermission is coming. Of course, I have to go to the bathroom. I am a 65-year-old male. So I nudge my wife, she knowingly says, "Go ahead. I'll meet you back here." I hop up in the dark, relearn how to walk and head to the appointment scheduled by my kidneys.

In this particular venue the bathroom situation is odd. Someone decided to put a drinking fountain between the male and female restrooms without considering all possible outcomes. The picture I see is the men's room on the left, the women's on the right and the drinking fountain in the middle. As I leave the restroom, I observe that the crowd has not arrived yet, so I quickly get a drink of water.

I hear the sound of a crowd massing just outside my vision. I know this is the "charge of the women." The light brigade had no clearer purpose than this sudden tsunami. Neither they nor I know what's about to happen.

I turn toward my right from the drinking fountain, inadvertently blocking the entrance to the ladies room. Suddenly I was faced with the lead lady of the small bladder. I immediately froze in place. Her panicked eyes stared at me urgently. I'm almost 6 feet 2 inches, and she is 5 feet 6 inches. My hands shake uncontrollably as I focus on stepping out of her way. But I'm frozen in place. There is now a growing pile-up of quick-stepping women maneuvering like cars at an off ramp on the LA freeway behind the leading lady. The women behind her flash urgent looks and utter demanding sounds.

I manage to sputter out, "Parkinson's. Frozen."

The lead woman starts to step around me to her left but suddenly halts when she realizes my hands are shaking at exactly the same level as her breasts. The crowd continues to build. Our eyes meet. She seems to be contemplating the trade-off between being accidentally fondled and wetting her pants.

My eyes must have said, "I'm not a weirdo." At least I hope they do. I try to stop my hands from gyrating while at the same time organize myself to a step out of her way. This can be done. We are both about to be crushed as the women in the sixth row back move forward as though the building behind them had caught fire.

Miraculously someone touches me on the right shoulder, breaking my concentration, and I step to my right. The unmolested woman charges forward, and the others pass by me in a strange sequence. The first few understood what they saw. Those who could not see as well give me looks which sequentially escalated from "What the hell was this all about?" to "If I didn't have to go so badly, I would cut you into chopped liver."

The miraculous someone whispers in my ear, "Had this concert been the Grateful Dead, that's what you would have been: the Gratefully Dead." It's my wife. "Are we done here?"

"Yes," I reply.

"How about getting a latte, double decaf?"

At that point she knows my heart cannot go back to pacing the Komodo drummers any longer. Don't you love it when someone you have been married to for 30 years or more just knows when you've had "enough?"

Chapter 16
Fly Fishing in a Small World

The fly line zinged by my right ear on its way to the rising brown trout 70 feet in front of me. As the line hit its full extension, the leader popped and the gray crane fly floated up, hovering for a second inches off the water. The water exploded as the brown took the fly in the air before having to compete with its powerful companions holding their place in the current. The fishing guide managing the drift boat exclaimed, "You nailed that one!"

As I set the hook, the guide deftly turned the boat so that I could begin the half an hour of sheer excitement where I tested my line and rod management skills against the bag of tricks this 5-pound brown trout had used many times to outwit anglers from around the world. The fish, of course, did not know at this point that I was going to release it to fight another day. It acted as though this was the end. I thought ahead of the fish, maintaining tension on the line so I didn't lose out to it and its finely honed survival tactic: "Surprise! I'm going the direction you didn't prepare for."

As the light danced off the water, my multitasking mind experienced the wonderful feeling that said, "I'm here, still able to do this." At the same time, my subconscious third eye seemed to look from above me, sensing that I was near my end of days of fly fishing. I was really here this time because of the generosity and friendship of someone who included the sense that it's all too much for him to experience alone in his passion for fishing. He made sure others had the opportunity to join in on the secrets anglers experience and share only with those who fish. My Parkinson's had progressed to the point where if I didn't have substantial support and someone to watch my back, I clearly could not have gone on a remote fishing trip like this. I needed the cooperation of those who found in themselves the desire for others to be there with them despite physical disabilities.

My excitement was broken suddenly by a sense of fatigue as my arms shook and my legs began to freeze up, putting a strain on my back. The trout sensed the moment and executed an arching jump, sweeping its tail across the line to twist out of the tension and was gone like a flash of lightning. The line zinged back toward me.

"They sense everything through that line." The guide observed. "It always amazes me."

"Yeah it's hard to hide the Parkinson's; so what's the upside?" I responded.

The other guy in the boat who was sipping a beer smiled and said, "What was that little story about hope springs eternal you told us last night?"

I gave his question a quick thought and repeated the story for the guide. "It's like Sven and Ole coming to the surface of the lake after their float plane loaded with their giant quartered moose crashes. Sven says to Ole, 'We got a little further than last year, Ole.'

"Ole replies, 'Yeah, we're getting the hang of it.'" At that point I looked back at the guy who was smiling broadly. "You mean I played this one longer than the last one that got away?"

"Yup, that's right on target for you today," the guide said. "Now I need you to explain again why it was Main

Street and Wall Street, which both operated using perverse incentives, created the bubble in the housing and financial markets."

I just shook my head. The other guy handed me a cold beer. This had been a fairly strange relationship. The guide was a very bright young man in his 30s who had managed to figure out how to get me to relax by continuously asking me questions about the current economic crisis. Then I was able to overcome the shake of Parkinson's and successfully cast my fly line. He'd found out I was an economist because his partner had been a student of mine. He told me he had a guest tomorrow who was a former member of the president's Cabinet who talked a lot about policy. My guide didn't want to be uninformed. I found his approach to getting me to fish to be curious, but it worked for me. Obviously, he had a sense of pride that made me like him even more than I would have based just on his skill in the business of managing to put anglers in the right place on the river to catch these magnificent fish.

Hearing thrashing sounds of someone almost jumping into the river, we both looked up.

"How often do you see guys do that?" I asked.

"Almost never," the guide smiled and said. "Your friend not only loves to play the fish, he likes to get in the water with the fish and move with the water. He's on the fish's turf and out of his own comfort zone. Not many guys do that." He added "Please don't you try that; I don't think I could get you back in the boat."

"Don't worry." I replied. "My comfort zone is right here in this boat."

We floated by my friend who was up to his armpits in the water, puffing on his cigar and playing the fish very carefully.

"You know you're about an inch away from disaster," I casually mentioned.

He laughed. "Yeah, this brown is smart."

The guide and I both knew nothing would happen to ruin this magic moment for this guy and his fish. Some things you just know. What was really going on among three separate people was the politics of human interaction where we each observe those around us, act on what we understand and work with the convergence of our interests to make our lives more than the sum of the parts. This positive sum became a memorable day for each person instead of an unlucky day where each person spent the time worrying about his issues alone. I could've been fretting about losing fish I hooked because of my Parkinson's symptoms. The guide could've been worrying that he was going to be out of his depth the next day. My friend could have been concerned that he was being a procrastinator. Instead, being together with the right attitude made it one of the lucky days.

I suddenly remembered and finished a thought. "Yeah those perverse incentives wouldn't have worked if it hadn't been for the fact that the Fed was pushing liquidity into the market at such low interest rates that all that money poured into that single market, driving prices wildly upward."

"So the money got into the market by people borrowing against their houses at inflated prices, and that's why that market bubbled," the guide replied. His answer was right on the money.

I relaxed happily hearing someone who wasn't going to take a test on the material become excited about it. But I guess that's not exactly true, his test was maintaining credibility when dealing with someone he obviously wanted to treat him with respect.

We moved on down to another of the guide's favorite spots. I knew the cycle would repeat itself, putting me very much at ease and allowing me to feel the motion of casting and the anticipation of that fly popping at the end of the line.

"You had a great teacher; when you are relaxed your casting motion has an old-style rhythm, much like my grandfather's," my guide said.

In my estimation he moved up a notch. "Thanks. My dad taught me. He would've been old enough to be your grandfather. It was the style of the time."

The day proceeded ahead, detached from the rest of the world, with its rhythm driven by the humming of the fly lines, the splash of the fish and the buzzing of the hatch. Receding in my mind was the thought that these days were among the last I could enjoy as the Parkinson's progressed. What I marveled at was the way in which we three provided each other the necessary counterpoint so that each of us could take care of important needs. I could still cast like it was 30 years ago, the guide could prepare to hold his own and my friend could feel that his love for fishing carried over to those beyond himself.

About two years after that day, on the way to my lifelong learning class on campus, I was stopped by an attorney I had known for many years. He was one of those attorneys whose style was defined by a constant cross examination of the world. Most people deduced that he simply was driven to make sure he knew everything he possibly could "just in case." No one really knew what case he was preparing for and neither did he. But he was driven.

"I hear you have an old-style flawless fly casting technique," he said.

"Where would you hear that?" I asked. I was taken aback since I did not imagine this lawyer would have any idea about my fly fishing life.

He smiled. He must have felt he had the advantage for the moment. "I was down in Chile and ran into one of our alumni."

This further confused me, but I was on the hook for more. He was playing me like a trout, and I knew it. "Okay, so what's the rest of the story?"

He kind of smiled, raised his chin and spoke slowly. "This alumni is a fishing guide and wanted to thank you for getting him prepared to hold his own with the bigwig politician he took fishing on the Beaverhead."

The pieces came together in my mind, and it was a great pleasure to know that it had all worked out. Having surprised someone with that tidbit of information he had gathered and effectively used for a moment of fun, the lawyer said goodbye and walked away with a little bounce in his step. In this fashion, he proved once again his theory that knowing everything is the key to enjoying the small pleasures of life, namely having the upper hand, even for a second.

I walked away thanking him in my mind for bringing me back to that day and for letting me know I'd been able to repay the gift the guide had given me by distracting me from my Parkinson's symptoms and putting me at ease. The encounter also provided a way for the lawyer to virtually join us on the trip, making the world a smaller place and bringing us all together again.

Relationship building is the extension of the self into the common space. This allows someone with Parkinson's to give something in exchange for the common good and "make their day." This is a great substitute for a "make my day" approach to relationships that gives no ground. The day of fishing joy would not have happened without the generosity of my friend who never got out of his depth. We all need to get close to our limits in order to experience the possible. I'm still fly fishing, but I wade the stream only up to my ankles. I'm not crazy!

Chapter 17
"I Can't Walk Just Now; Could You Please Get Me That Bicycle?"

As I have discussed before, one of the more vexing problems facing each person dealing with Parkinson's is the problem explaining the "off" and "on" states that he or she will transition through in a given day, or maybe even in a few hours, or perhaps even in minutes. The problem itself has both good and bad aspects. The good aspect is that when I'm "on" that means my medicine is working, and I appear nearly normal. Within a given period of time, in my case after 12 years, two and one half to three hours may pass before suddenly I'm "off." When I'm "off" my body will exhibit freezing, slowness of gait, flat affect and smaller voice, small writing and tremors in my hands and sometimes my legs. To the outside world, it is virtually inexplicable how I could go from one state to the other without being hit by a car or falling off a building. I have even had people ask me if I had a stroke. My normal response is "Not since you last saw me an hour (a day) ago." That usually takes the tension out of the moment. They laugh and say something like, "Of course, so what's going on?" At that point I try to engage in some sort of explanation and bring them up to speed as best I can on Parkinson's. Being "on" then "off" is probably the least difficult of public situations.

The more difficult situation arises when I am "off" yet still able to do such things as ride a bicycle, swim, drive or play golf. This situation can lead people to believe I'm faking. It undermines credibility if they are not given some information to help them understand the issues. As it turns out the situation is deeply rooted in the biochemistry of Parkinson's.

At the biochemical level, Parkinson's symptoms by and large arise due to the death of dopamine producing cells in the substantia nigra part of the brain. The substantia nigra is a small region in the brain stem which helps control movement. Its cells produce dopamine, which assists other brain cells in their functions. When this process malfunctions, it causes loss of physical control, tremors and rigidity that is common in Parkinson's.

Parkinson's seems not to affect those motor responses that are fully autonomic like heartbeat, but primarily affects those that are subliminal that, over time, have become pretty automatic. It does not substantially affect those motor responses that are classically overt such as riding a bicycle, swinging a golf club or swimming until the final stages of PD. This is particularly true in my case. I have talked with others who experience the same phenomenon. This three-way division is even more difficult to explain, particularly when dealing with a new acquaintance or someone involved at a point in time when the old body chemistry is changing from "on" to "off."

I recall an afternoon a few summers ago where I went down to the pool at our townhouse on Flathead Lake. I walked down like a normal human being in my bathing suit with a towel, hat and sunglasses. The day was magnificent. The sky was crystal clear cobalt blue, the lake shimmering in the light and a bald eagle was busy fishing in the bay. I went down and took some time to swim a few laps in the pool as fast as I could to get my heart rate up, stretch my muscles and just enjoy a swim in 80 degree water instead of our more common 60 degree swim from the boat in the lake.

It turns out my timing was a little bit off. As I got out of the pool, I could tell that I was transitioning from "on" to "off." Being about 150 yards and two minutes from the townhouse where I could take the medicine which would return me to my "on" state, I realized I was in a bit of a self-made predicament. About 30 feet from the pool the "off" symptoms began to present themselves. First my steps became shorter, and my posture began to bend forward. Very quickly I was walking with a shuffling gait, stopping every eight to 12 steps, freezing up and then taking 20 to 30 seconds to initiate the next step.

One of my neighbors was down at the pool as well. I could tell he'd never seen this phenomenon before when he said, "Are you okay? Are you having a heart attack or stroke or something?" Not only was he alarmed, he was 90 years old and in failing health.

I did not reveal to him that I was suddenly more concerned about his level of agitation than my problems.

Being the good soul he was, he began to come over to help me across an area of round stones that some people thought were decorative but I knew were mostly dangerous because they were loose and treacherous.

"Oh my God," I thought. "He's going to fall and break his hip. When people show up, I'll be 'on' again, and he will be injured." Most importantly, I wouldn't be able to get to him quickly when he fell which I knew was about to happen. My brain began to engage, and I looked around. I spotted a bicycle leaning against the pool house. If I could coax him through the stones, he was only about 12 feet from the bicycle.

"I can't walk just now, could you please get me that bicycle," I said.

Well, that achieved one of my goals. He stopped dead in his tracks. "What? How is that going to help?" he asked.

"No stroke, no heart attack just my Parkinson's acting up," I said. "I'll be fine as long as you don't fall down in those rocks."

At that point, he realized that he made a mistake in his Good Samaritan move by getting out in those rocks. He quickly and very carefully moved out of the rocks and grabbed the handle bars of the bicycle.

He smiled from ear to ear. "Okay I'll walk it over to you."

I thanked him profusely and patted him on the back when he delivered the bicycle.

"Well that got me off my ass," He said with an ironic tone.

"At least you didn't fall on your ass," I responded.

We both laughed.

"So where do we go from here?" he asked.

I thought for a second. "I need to get my meds," I said. "Why don't you sit by the pool for a few minutes while I get over this 'off' state, and I'll drive you back to your place in my golf cart?"

"That's all good and well, but how are you going to get back to your place and get back here before I get sunburned as slow as you're walking?" At 90, he was still sharp as a tack.

"Just like this." I chuckled and slowly threw my leg over the bicycle and rode off laughing.

"Well I'll be damned."

To me he sounded like W.C. Fields. I was the kid who'd pestered and annoyed him — the kid the old actor had once told, "Go away. You draw flies."

I quickly took my meds, made my transition from bicycle to golf cart and picked him up. As I dropped him back at his townhouse, he asked in sort of a bemused way, "How did you do that?" I explained what I knew to him over the next few minutes, and we ended the conversation with his reflection on it all.

He looked puzzled but happy and summed it all up as follows, "I'll be a monkey's uncle. You can learn something every day." At 90 he knew a lot.

These kinds of transitions are not always so smooth and enjoyed with such wonderful company. But I did feel that bringing him up to speed with how Parkinson's works got me a new recruit for the cause. That's how understanding develops: one person at a time.

Chapter 18
"I'll Get You up the Stairs!"

"I'll get you up the stairs!" A shockingly loud voice broke my concentration.

"At least she didn't say sweetie!" This was my first thought as I resisted her attempt to lift me up the first step.

I had just entered the hotel after a long car trip, and I was on my way upstairs to relax. Now, I was in the grip of someone who was going to help me whether I needed it or not. I did not. I had just stumbled over to the steps on my way up to the room after a four hour drive. I was trying to use steps as opposed to the elevator as my way of getting back in contact with my legs. At 65, even if I didn't have Parkinson's, my legs could still go to sleep on a four-hour torturous drive through New Mexico.

My wife and I were on a trip coming down from Breckenridge, Colorado to Albuquerque, passing through the high Rockies down into the San Luis Valley and stopping along the way to do some research for a book I was writing. That had gone well. But we discovered that with my Parkinson's, we seemed to be able to travel about 80 miles during a day before I just wore out. This last day's drive of 120 miles was more than I was prepared for, but I made it. I was now ready for a good sleep before we flew back home in the morning.

When a person is "off" with Parkinson's, the world is a very different place than when a person is "on." One of the most striking elements of that difference is the relationship between gravity and the space through which a person has to move. In my case, and the case of many others I've spoken with regarding this issue, stairs are actually a friend.

An open expanse of flat floor, such as in a museum, tricks the brain in two ways. The first is accomplished by perspective which makes a flat floor appear to rise away from the observer. The second is that many different kinds of marble, tile and polished wood look like ice or at least slick wet surfaces. These combined effects on the brain cause the brain confusion, making a flat floor look like ice on an incline. The brain infers from this information that imminent danger lies ahead, initiating a do-not-step response to avoid slipping and falling. This creates anxiety which generates a sensation of operating in three dimensions. All movement options seem equally dangerous to the Parkinson's brain. Thus no option seems possible without falling.

This form of unresolvable choice has to be overcome in order to walk normally. That is why a sudden distraction can break the spell of indecision in the Parkinson's brain, allowing the possibility of a first step, and then another to take place and allow semi-normal walking to resume.

It is very much like the feeling many people have when they first learn to ski, where they must learn that the only security they have from falling is to lean downhill, a counter intuitive move. Those who lean back toward the hill soon find themselves racing down out of control, doing the opposite of what they wanted.

Stairs, however, involve no control of perception. At first glance, it is easy to see that they go up or down. Anyone able to get to the stairs will be able to feel gravity's clarifying force when considering going up or down. To negotiate stairs is simple — just step up or step down. The feeling is one of two dimensions rather than three. Of course, with stairs there is usually a handrail. That aid is not available in an open floor space adding that third dimension. In fact I've often mentioned to others, that if I had the perfect house, I would have it designed by Escher with continuous stairways. They are initially puzzled, but soon understand my point, an epiphany.

The general public, and in this case the specific slightly inebriated woman I dealt with that day, does not understand the movement issues people with PD have. If one is impaired, people generally assume that steps are a problem. That is, in part, because when they see disabled people having difficulties stumbling around on the flat floor, the unknowing person believes stairs would be even more challenging. This is why the PD impaired person gets lots of offers of help dealing with steps and less commonly on flat floors. This help on stairs is often more destructive than helpful. When I am moving up or down stairs, and someone grabs an arm, suddenly there are too many points of contact. The brain equalizes weight to all points and the only safe move is to stop. This is frustrating because moving, even on stairs, can be difficult to initiate. The sudden unwanted help destroys my small victory over being frozen.

It would be more helpful if the bystander waited to respond to a request for assistance than to barge in with too much too soon.

So what is the proper thing to do when you are in the grip of a slightly inebriated "good Samaritan" who has just made it impossible to continue moving forward or to go up or down the stairs?

The mind says, "Let go of me!" The mouth utters, "Thank you, I'll be okay," while a tense smile breaks out. Most people let go, slightly inebriated people do not.

"Are you brain injured?" the woman asked.

Someone with an injured brain would say, "Yes," as if

brain injury was a communicable disease. My healthy brain informed me, "I do not want to talk about Parkinson's now."

"No," I told her.

"Don't be sensitive, it takes time to get over being hit on the head," she said.

My mind focused on the effects of alcohol on judgement. Finally the point of no return had arrived.

"I do not have a brain injury. Thank you. I do not want any help. I'm trying to manage on my own because it helps me remain independent given my walking problems."

"Well, goody for you. I'm not needed, so where was I going?" she asked no one in particular.

I offered some help. "I don't know, but it seemed like you were heading out the door."

In my thoughts, I quietly disengaged from this awkward moment and, trudging upwards, thought about sleep.

"The bags are in the room," my wife said from the top of the stairs. Then she whispered, "Well it didn't take a long time to deal with her."

"For once I avoided having to explain Parkinson's and that sped up getting free." I mumbled.

My wife touched my arm and in a soft voice purred, "I love you. You're learning how to deal with it."

"Which?" I asked. "The Parkinson's or well-meaning people doing the wrong thing?"

"Both."

Chapter 19
"I Used to Walk Like That, but I'm Over It Now"

If a person has Parkinson's and has tried and succeeded in developing a strategy that makes him or her feel self-actualized and managing their situation effectively, then the person has realized a major achievement in life. The problem with that level of success is losing sight of some of its underpinnings. Recalling that successful management of Parkinson's requires both an internal and external balancing of awareness so the proper tactic is used to manage the imminent challenge, losing track of that balance can lead to some problems in dealing with the outside world. Careful observation is very important for success in personal encounters. Disabled people, in general, don't always appear competent. So they have to guard against the opportunist intruding on their freedom of action or becoming the object of harassment if they become isolated or marginalized in some fashion.

This can happen especially when a Parkinson's sufferer has become frozen halfway out a door, is fighting the spring in the door or is unable to initiate a step appearing hunched over with their walking stick tapping on the floor. The person with Parkinson's is trapped in this situation and appears unable to get out of the predicament. In fact, he or she is looking around to see if a spot on the floor can be identified, providing a possible target that would allow a crucial first step. It is called target walking. Although it makes perfect sense to the person with Parkinson's, to the observer the person looks like a candidate for residency at a nursing home. Soon!

A couple of years ago I was at a restaurant with some friends having a very nice time enjoying a lovely dinner with great views of a spectacular sunset. As I was returning from the every half an hour walk I try to take during social events, especially when I'm sitting down a lot, I got stuck in the doorway to the deck. Not only did I block the main entrance, I also blocked the hallway to the bathroom.

Fortunately, nobody was moving through the area so I proceeded with my attempt at target walking. This involved picking a spot out front of my foot to step toward to try to initiate walking out of the freezing position. Once I found it, I let go of the spring-loaded door creating somewhat of a great crashing sound.

As I reacted to the noise, a person rushed by me. I continued to walk forward, stumbling on my toes, lurching forward, just to keep my momentum going.

"I used to walk like that, but I'm over it now," a young man stated rather abruptly. He was imitating my walking and seemingly mocking my situation.

"That's inappropriate behavior. Let's talk for a second."

I may have been overly sensitive.

Part of my tactical approach to these situations is to deal directly with the person in a non-hostile but clear approach which I view as a teaching moment. This generally works very well, but in this case the young man just kept going around the corner into the bar. I certainly wasn't chasing him down, but it did upset me.

However, it was enough of a distraction to allow me to

slip into a normal walking gait. This type of agitating distraction, which often heightens brain activity and adrenaline levels, has had the effect of stopping symptomatic problems on a number of occasions. This isn't exactly how I want my situation to improve, but sometimes a person takes what he can get. So I entered the bar walking pretty normally.

"You're better now, Sir," a voice to my right and slightly out of my vision commented.

I stopped and turned. "Thanks, but I..."

My little speech came to an abrupt end as I looked at the speaker. The young man looking back into my eyes had Down's syndrome. I clearly sputtered.

"My boy says he was helping out with your walking problem," the young man's broadly smiling father said to me.

Talk about having to quickly reorient. I felt like I was on black ice and had just decided to make a U-turn. Major sliding going on and corrective measures being sought very rapidly described my mental condition. I blurted out the next thought. "I was stumbling. I have Parkinson's."

"You could fall down," The young man responded.

Whereupon I collected myself and simply stated, "You're right. Thanks for breaking my concentration. That's what I was really worried about."

"Worrying about falling is the worst isn't it?" he said to his dad.

"Yeah, we solved that problem a long time ago didn't we?" his father said with a smile.

"Yeah, Dad," the young man said as he and his dad seemed to lean closer together, creating a kind of comfort zone.

I thanked them both and moved on, thinking to myself how important it is to clearly understand a situation before applying a standard approach to dealing with it. It's rare that a misperception will be this obvious. There was no misunderstanding. What I had just learned was a helpful lesson for me and a positive reflection on humanity. These two guys knew how to solve problems and were trying to be helpful. Like me they were a little rough around the edges.

Chapter 20
"Do One Thing a Year that Is Scary; You'll Live Longer"

When I was being strapped up and snapped on to a zip line running a mile or so in 12 stages through the Costa Rican forest canopy, the following thought came into my mind: "I always tell everybody that my wife always demonstrates good judgment."

After she'd scheduled the zip line tour, I had looked at her in some bemusement and asked, "What were you thinking?"

"We're adopting a new philosophy," she replied.

"Zip lining is a philosophy?"

She laughed. "No, its best summed up by an idea that popped into my mind the other day."

What I didn't say was, "You mean when you started to twitch during the boring seminar we were attending on retirement and health management?" What I did say was, "Were you drinking alone?"

She gave me a look that indicated that I should not have said what I thought. She smiled broadly and said, "No." With a little wink she announced that we should live by the following motto, "Do one thing a year that's scary; you'll live longer."

"Who gave you that advice?" I quipped.

"It was my own inspiration." She laughed again.

Zip lining in Costa Rica — just scary enough.

"Remember right hand on the lower cable, left-hand on the strap." A voice broke into my thought process and suddenly, whir! I was off, heading down the cable. In the first two feet you're committed, and I was 10 feet down the cable. A huge smile crossed my face as I realized that this adventure was truly inspired.

As I gained speed, I felt a bit of heat through the heavy leather glove on my right hand. I realized that in the last couple of years we had become more and more cautious because of the weakening effect of my medicine on my Parkinson's symptoms. I was now 12 years out from diagnosis and eight to nine years out from the use of levodopa/carbidopa as my primary medicine. Any doctor worth visiting will tell you that this levodopa/carbidopa medicine, which allows your body to synthesize dopamine, seems to wear out after six or seven years as PD progresses.

In fact, four months before I began my zip line adventure the medicine essentially stopped working. This caused a great deal of upset since my symptoms were full-blown and out of control for about a month and a half until my wonderful neurologist devised a plan to keep that medicine going and add one that was relatively new in the FDA arsenal. This magical cocktail returned my body to a fairly normal state for someone who'd been living with Parkinson's for 12 years. With great relief, it also allowed me to put the deep brain stimulation (DBS) surgery out of immediate consideration.

The idea that without risk high rewards are hard to come by is a concept well known to economists and financial investors. It, also, is true when applied to many of life's choices. In the first eight years of my Parkinson's we continued to do the things we had always done, including downhill skiing, swimming in the ocean and in large lakes, sea kayaking, biking and cross-country skiing in mountainous terrain.

The only specific accommodation we had made was to replace scuba diving with snorkeling. In part this was simply safer for the Parkinson's afflicted person and for a person's diving buddy and other divers you might be with. As far as I know it's not required by PADI diving safety recommendations, but it makes sense.

My wife and I recall with some terror hearing about a woman who had failed to tell the dive master she had heart problems. (Although one might have been suspicious of someone carrying about 300 pounds and looking about 55 years old.) She and her much smaller husband went scuba diving, and at 30 feet below the surface she had a massive coronary and expired. They could not lift her into the dive boat so she had to be lashed to the starboard side of the boat and taken back to the dock in full view of all the dive boats going out.

Our dive master told us the story as a cautionary tale and knowing I was an economist and my wife, a marketer, he wanted to know how bad this sight might have been for business.

Our response was, "Not so good," spoken in unison.

We made minor to major adjustments in our other activities as my endurance decreased, which was partially attributable to Parkinson's and partly to aging. We also had to learn to carefully prepare so that "on" times coincided with activity planning. If "off" symptoms appeared, we had to be ready to get to a safe place, take the medicine required and wait until I was back "on." What actually occurred was our trips became increasingly short. I felt that the only thing really keeping me going was the fact I continued to play handball about three times a week throughout this time.

One distinct aspect of continuing each of these activities was an odd phenomenon that began to occur for me in virtually every sporting, risk-taking activity I continued to engage in. It was a phenomenon I called "joining up." Much like a horse whose confidence you have won will come up to you in the corral, not looking for food but ready for some activity, I would constantly be joined by people while I was skiing, biking or, in this case, zip lining, who would stay with me for a while or for the rest of the day. After a period of introductory conversation and the general open friendliness one finds in these situations, it would inevitably turn out that they had a loved one with Parkinson's or some movement disorder. I continued to operate under the delusion that when I was "on" I looked normal. Apparently, the shaking and awkwardness that remained in every activity such as making great left ski turns and then wildly strange right ones gave me away.

The joining up usually began with the following question, "How you doing?" My response was typically, "I'm just fine, how are you on this gorgeous day?"

(Did I mention that we began to restrict ourselves to being only fair weather participants in sporting activities? Avoiding bad weather is the major safety move in many of the activities we planned.)

I realized if I wasn't out here doing this, I would not have the opportunity to meet these people. In every case, it turned out to be exactly right. After the normal pleasantries and the typical "Who are you and where are you from?" conversation sprinkled with, "What do you do or what did you used to do?" the conversation inevitably went to, "How do you do this with Parkinson's?"

The typical answer was, "I really can only do it when I'm 'on.'" This was usually followed by a quick discussion of what "on" and "off" meant in my case. "On" was not really a situation where no symptoms exist. I've discussed this with numerous neurologists and received no specific or precise answer from them.

My answer to the question about how I could do one

thing and not another was as truthful as I could make it. "I don't really know how I can do one thing such as ski when at the same time I would be unable to walk normally."

This is the truth for me and many, many Parkinson's sufferers I've talked with over the past 12 years. All I can really say is that I'm sure being "on" has to do with the fact that I have kept exercising, and only resorted to walking sticks, wheelchairs and other aides when I simply cannot move or have to move quickly in airports. For the people I deal with, some find this bizarre because they see me walking or doing some fairly physical activity one time, and at another time see that I am hardly moving or am frozen with a walking stick in my hand.

After this discussion, the person who has initiated the joining up process understands I don't need protection and is ready to move forward with the discussion. Very frequently they next ask me why I am taking risks associated with skiing, biking or zip line aerobatics. Some treat me like I am crazy, others in a helpful way, give the impression they think I am in denial. Finally those who shake their heads realize that I am still trying to live a full rich life. I'm quite sure they are all correct.

Some years ago I was skiing very badly down a black diamond ski run, no longer bouncing and twisting and turning with some rhythm, I fell hard. Within a moment, two guys skied over. They each grabbed me by an arm and lifted me back up and rather impolitely announced, "Are you crazy? You shouldn't be skiing on this run."

"I thought I was doing pretty well until I fell," I said.

They quickly corrected me. "No, you fell because you are not doing well, and if you look ahead very far, this run just gets meaner and meaner," the older one said shaking his head.

Some distant memory emerged. I recalled watching other skiers who were in over their heads, typically not knowing where they were going. In order to survive in the moment, they were looking straight down at their skis. Then, I remembered I had been looking straight down at my skis when I fell.

Now that I was standing up, my shaking hands drew their attention. The one in the cobalt blue ski suit said, "I'm a doc. It seems you have Parkinson's. We really can't go on and leave you here because on your next fall you're likely to go down the slope out of control like a turtle on its back."

"Gotcha," I said, following up as quickly as I could with, "I think I get the message."

They both nodded and dropped down below me to say goodbye. Their wives, whom I hadn't noticed yet, suddenly came into view. The brunette observed, "Good job, guys." Looking me in the eyes, she asked "Will we meet you down at the bar?"

"Sure, I'm buying."

"That's right, we'll all need it."

The four of them skied down the hill like I used to do while I side-hilled over to the nearest groomed blue run, chagrined but uninjured. We did meet at the bar. It did cost me $62.00, but they paid the tip and bought the nachos. My wife and a few friends came in looking for me, and unfortunately, they were able to discover through my new friends loose lips that I had in fact gone down a black diamond. My wife and friends were unresponsive to my protests that I had safely ended my skiing day on the blue run. The consensus was that I was still capable of learning, but my fantasy about my skill had to be purged.

"Keep skiing but don't keep the ski patrol busy," the doc said. It cost me another $37.00 for the next round with the combined group. Apparently rescue is more expensive than companionship.

These thoughts and memories rushed through my mind as I zip lined through the forest canopy, whizzing past howler monkeys who were so accustomed to crazy people that they paid no attention to us at all. My wife's inspired philosophy had gotten me here, but we had agreed that if I was in the "off" position, I would just wait in the bus with some cookies.

I was "off" for part of the trip from our hotel. This unnerved our guide, and he began to "join up" with my wife and me. By the time we were getting into our gear for the zip line, the three of us were chatting it up, and he was clearly assessing me minute by minute.

"I'll go last," I said.

He breathed a sigh of relief and added that my wife should go in front of me, and he would follow. This lineup held and in each of the 12 stations, which are little platforms lashed to trees 60 to 90 feet in the air. At each he made sure to check my progress.

No heroics were involved. The adrenaline rush was huge. Frankly, the rush seemed to prolong my "on" time. We all enjoyed the experience and the screaming delight of the teenagers in the group. He admitted that he was a bit uneasy about my condition at first but surprised at how the experience seemed to make me better as we went along. I explained that there was a new finding in exercise/Parkinson's research where Parkinson's sufferers who road fixed tandem bicycles with very athletic people at 90 RPMs for one hour three days a week for three weeks had substantial reduction in symptoms for the next five weeks. Often times the Parkinson's guinea pig was not really continuing to spin but was passively letting his legs relax and move at that speed. This is called "forced" exercise. Sort of what was happening to me on the zip line.

What seems to be happening is that when a person starts exercising the body, the brain thinks it's going to be operating at this extraordinarily high level and generates dopamine levels that may not match the level needed for the high-end exercise because of the Parkinson's, but will exceed what such a person would normally produce.

Our guide nodded thoughtfully at this idea and sort of

laughed. He stated that he thought I would be okay. He could take care of almost anything given his training. But he was worried about fatigue. He pulled out six or seven packages of M&Ms and a couple of weird Costa Rican candy bars from his pockets and said, "I guess I'll have to eat all these myself."

I can assure you he got a huge tip from me.

I don't know what next year holds. But I am confident that I will be tackling at least one risky adventure. I look forward to meeting whoever joins up for the next wild thing I do. Just as exercise tricks the brain, doing something scary tricked mine. I felt almost normal again.

Chapter 21
"These Are Not Real Tears"

A soft bong sound came from my computer. I was somewhere between "on" and "off," sort of in a daze waiting for my drugs to work their magic. I managed to get up, take a couple of shuffling steps, then a real step lurching forward to arrive in front of the computer. The new mail notice made my heart jump. I clicked on the sender's address, and there appeared this lovely little message:

"Hi Grammie and Den, it's me. Today I got an email account. I am so excited to come home and see you guys."

This was her first email ever. She was eight and reminded her mother that her older sister had received her email account when she turned eight. Siblings are very attentive to the timing of other siblings' progress toward adulthood.

This email from my granddaughter was meaningful by any standard but the effect on me was tears, a shaking lower lip and flushed red face, making me look and sound confused. This wonderful little moment fully unmasked one of the most unusual aspects of Parkinson's that I have had to deal with: the inability to control the expression of my emotions.

Well-adjusted adults typically have reached the point where they can usually control the ways in which they express their emotions. Fully functioning adults are capable of making their emotional expression convey their feelings to others both as genuine and as a part of their personal negotiation with others as they establish relationships among their family, friends and co-workers. These skills are very important. We develop relationships with others by skillful use of these emotional connections.

The failure to establish relationships often comes as a result of misunderstanding emotional expressions or being put off by the volatility of another person's emotions. Sometimes it simply is a difference in emotional expression between people that precipitates problems. With Parkinson's it is difficult to manage one's way through what is often an involuntary emotional minefield. Many times we can't control the level of physical expression our emotions generate. Such levels can exceed what is normal among well-adjusted adults.

The emotions of anger, sadness, joy and happiness are just a few broad categories of emotion that require fine tuning in complex adult relations. When Parkinson's is in full bloom, it is my experience that fine tuning becomes extremely difficult. The feeling is one of being unmasked. When an unexpected physical response occurs there is a sudden awareness that the expression of emotion, such as crying, is as much a surprise to me as it is to others, and it's difficult to control. My experience of tearing up as though someone dear to me died over this wonderful moment created by my lovely granddaughter was unnerving. The expression was completely out of control relative to the emotional place this event would usually have for me or anyone else.

If my granddaughter were present she might wonder if her granddad had "lost it" or maybe even think she shouldn't have sent the email since she'd wanted me to share in her happiness, and it wasn't happening. Eight-year-old youngsters are great judges of this inconsistency between intent and outcome.

It is likely to be ineffective to simply say, "These are not real tears." A person is left with either affirming that the loving act was too much, or that he or she is sort of out-of-control. These options are not very good for building a relationship with a granddaughter or any other person. It is easy to tell that emotions are expressing themselves in an out-of-control fashion when they are disproportionate to the situation. The risk is the possibility of pushing away loved ones and friends, let alone well-meaning strangers, as a result of this confusing response.

Fortunately, when this happened, my granddaughter was 5,000 miles away. But it reminded me how important it is for a person with Parkinson's to think through setting emotional expectations in advance of events. This insight really means being very candid when it is necessary to disclose lack of emotional control to others. PD is not an excuse. But it is the cause. I learned that it is important to convey that the emotion a person with Parkinson's has is as genuine as it would have been before Parkinson's, but now the expression of that emotion is not under control. It is self-awareness that makes one realize tears are flowing in the situation that normally wouldn't make one cry.

On the opposite end of the spectrum it is often observed that over time people afflicted with Parkinson's develop a flat affect. Flat affect basically means that there is little facial expression change when something is funny, sad, joyous or tragic.

I became aware of this primarily through my wife and family. There have been times when my wife will be laughing heartily, and she asks, "Why are you not laughing?"

This surprises me. I will often look puzzled because I think I am laughing when I am not. I believe something is lost from that wonderful sense of laughing with someone you feel in sync with. My wife and I have talked this through which allows me to be self-aware enough in some situations to overcome the Parkinson's tendency to not express emotion. I would call this tunnel vision. I counteract this "tunnel vision," for example, by watching television as though I were driving down a busy street. I tend to keep looking around the room away from the television in a sort of search pattern. When we have guests for a movie or to watch some sporting event, I occasionally catch friends looking around the room with me wondering if I'm looking for invading rodents or yellow jackets. Most people when they hear my explanation usually say something like, "Oh yeah that makes sense," with that tone of voice that implies acceptance, but not understanding.

Anger, on the hand, is much more complicated than humor. I recall a situation where I was staying with family in Europe, and an unexpected accident occurred. In this situation I was being treated, as always, with gracious hospitality. The breakfast table was set as if my wife and I were visiting royalty. The home was an elegant one where quality art and craftsmanship was everywhere to be enjoyed. Unfortunately, my shaking and unstable movement caused me to feel a bit like a bull in a China shop. My response to this was to be extraordinarily careful which led to taking a very long time to get to the dining room table. I may have been mistaken, but as I approached, I didn't hear anyone breathe.

After I sat down and joined the wonderful ceremony of breakfast, everything seemed to be going smoothly until I decided to pour myself some orange juice. Unfortunately, in mid-pour my hand gyrated. I dropped the glass breaking what I knew was an antique and possibly a, "no replacement available" glass. I was profoundly angry at myself for forgetting that pouring was no longer in my skill set.

There was a moment of quiet, then a bustle of activity

where the juice was cleaned up, the glass shards vanished and a new and different glass appeared full of orange juice. The situation could not have been handled with more grace, but I found that I was unable to express myself. I know my face appeared indifferent; I was anything but. My anger at my error was so overwhelming that my wife intervened to help express my regrets for the disaster I caused.

Of course, our hosts were understanding and realized that my regret over the incident was genuine. But I felt ineffective in expressing myself clearly. In my mind I knew that my response could be interpreted as casual. It was some time before I convinced myself that I had adequately dealt with the situation. If ever there were an example of the ability of people to overlook my clumsiness, this was it. I will never forget being told by my hosts that my apology was unnecessary because, "the destruction of one glass makes the remaining glasses rarer and probably increases their value."

Sometimes Parkinson's can cause people to cry when they're not sad, other times to show no emotion when happy or angry. These are confusing signals to others and confounding to the person with PD. Lack of understanding about how Parkinson's interferes with the expression of emotions can create the wrong impressions. In these cases, the tears may be absolutely real.

Chapter 22
Tap, Tap, Tap: Keeping Time with Walking Sticks

I never imagined I would find myself unable to control my arms, my shoulder movements and the twisting of my torso. My way of dealing with these issues is to always let it happen normally with no apologies and with a straightforward composure. I get a lot of space to operate in when I golf. Not so much around the house or in large crowds.

The tapping of a walking stick is an activity that creates a response from people. In my case I typically walk with a walking stick when I'm "off." That's fine on rugs, but hardwood floors and marble floors become a bit of a nemesis. Since my hand is shaking, the walking stick tends to go tap, tap, tap on the hard flooring. This represents many things to many people. My grandchildren are happy that I can no longer sneak up on them anymore for a quick tickle. At least that's what they say as they come after me to get the tickling going. Turnabout is fair play.

My wife is happy I'm moving, but the walking stick keys into a very unpleasant memory of the stern Mrs. Fifi, her ballet teacher when she was young. Mrs. Fifi kept time to the music by pounding her staff on the floor. It seems the more the ballerinas failed to meet her standards of rhythm or execution the louder the tapping would become. This made a deep impression on my wife who actually became a professional singer/dancer. Yet, she never forgot those early traumatic days when the tap, tap, tap increased in intensity the more errors she made. Obviously, no husband wants to awaken that memory so I find myself taking the rug routes in the house as often as possible to avoid disturbing my wife's psyche.

Obviously, movement issues and the use of a walking stick are not confined to those with Parkinson's. One aspect, however, is relatively more common with Parkinson's and that is the phenomenon of freezing, being unable to initiate the next step. This strange behavior occurs with no warning and in no particular place with the possible exception of its frequent occurrence in doorways. When using a walking stick that is bouncing on the floor to the rhythm of a Parkinson's tremor, I appear not as disabled when freezing, but as a real hazard or annoyance. One of the really difficult side effects that comes with Parkinson's is that increased stress causes the freezing to get more pronounced. It also speeds up the walking stick floor tapping rate. I become Ms. Fifi.

Outside the home environment, I find the effect of the tapping of walking sticks can becomes more complex.

Some years ago, upon arrival at the Zürich International Airport I was tired, stiff and frankly very Parky after a nonstop flight from Minneapolis. We found ourselves in a hyper race through an airport that's roughly the size of Luxembourg. After what must have been six escalators and half a mile of clean, white tunnels, security and passport control we arrived at a huge light rail station. We and 875 others descended on the station because three flights had been scheduled to arrive simultaneously.

We stood around impatiently waiting for the train to arrive. I was in a dilemma. If I stood where the train doors were destined to open in my current state, I was likely to block the 875 people behind me when the train arrived, and I was frozen in place.

If I waited until they all were at the doors of the train, then I would likely miss the train, since I was unable to move fast enough to follow them and avoid being caught in the automatic doors.

The strategic move was clearly to move all the way to the left of the crowd, about midway between the doors and the majority of the passengers behind me. From there I would move on the fringe toward the first door once the train arrived, hopefully getting through before I got squashed. What would happen if I made the train's cyber voice jump into its high-pitched message: "Please clear the door now! The train is leaving"? As I took my position, my anxiety rose to a crescendo. The air mass in front of me stirred ahead of the train's arrival. The result was that the tapping of my walking stick on the marble floor grew from little taps to full jackhammer. People around me, who already endured enough annoyances on the trip, began glancing at me, shushing me and generally acting annoyed.

The doors opened and off we went. They rush-walked, and I tap-shuffled being bumped side to side and pushed from behind. The announcement that the doors were shutting caught me three perilous steps short. Panic had to be avoided. The man in front to my left stepped in front of me and said, "Grab my shoulder." I did, banging his head with my walking stick, and we were suddenly in the train with the door squeezed tightly behind me.

"Thanks," I said as he disappeared into the crowd.

"That was a nice move on his part despite the shot to his head," the fellow next to me observed, giving me the international "It's okay" nod.

I smiled pitifully. My wife peered through the sandwiched bodies between us and asked, "Are you okay?"

I smiled. Now where could I buy some soft foam to

wrap both ends of my walking stick, since it had gotten me into trouble? The train arrived at our destination and the press of people moved ahead of me, seemingly even more determined than ever to end the "flight arrival" nightmare.

My walking stick still reminds me of the differential impact-walking aids, including wheelchairs, have on the person using them and others. The phrase "can't live with 'em, can't live without 'em" comes to mind as I trudge and tap my way through life hoping that people generally know that my intentions are good.

Chapter 23
"I Don't Think Shaking It Will Fix It"

I had done virtually everything I could to get my timing under control. I was in a situation where I had a deadline on a federal court case for my final report, and the cartridge in my laser printer was not going to give me any more pages. I become irrational when computer systems don't obey. And I, of course, had heard rumors that these cartridges were set to run out after a certain number of pages even if they still had ink in them. I had shaken the cartridge and put it back in the printer. But it refused to do its job.

In retrospect I could have just put the report on a thumb drive and had it printed at my favorite print and copy stop. But I knew that the basic information in the case was changing, and I likely would have to revise the report overnight. Another trip up and down the canyon from my house first thing in the morning on our steep and icy roads was something I wanted to avoid if I could. Still, the deadline had to be met for filing with the court. So no matter what, I needed a new cartridge. As the reader can tell, this was some years ago before scanning, the use of attachments and PDFs made internet connectedness more flexible.

I managed to get to the computer store and parked my car at about a 9 degree angle on the snowdrift in the handicap parking space as close to the front door as possible. The cumulative effect of the stress of meeting the deadline, driving through a blizzard and stretching my medicine trying to extend my "on" condition meant I could sense "off" coming fairly quickly. I fumbled through my pills and took the next dosage about 45 minutes early. The combination of stress and heightened activity tends to speed up the use of the medicine much like going faster on the highway increases gas consumption. Sometimes one actually does feel like the tank is draining. The good news was that I'd taken the medicine and should be okay soon. The bad news was I felt "off" coming.

"Nearly normal" approaches being an oxymoron and can be very misleading. In this particular case I ignored the "you're about to be 'off'" warnings. I grabbed the bag holding the cartridge, got out of the car and headed toward the front door of the store. My hands began to shake, my legs stiffened up, my gate shortened and about thirty feet from the car and with two lanes of traffic to cross to get to the door, I froze. In Montana given the wind chill at about 25 degrees below zero that's literally possible, but in my case this was pure Parkinson's. I looked up and saw a car that was coming on my right nicely hit the brakes and slide to a stop. The driver's expression can only be described as "bug eyed."

I was not in his lane of traffic, but I was at the crosswalk so he had to stop. But why the emergency stop? Did he not see me? If he hadn't stopped, he would have run me over because by that time I would have been in his lane of traffic if everything was normal. Since I did freeze up, I guess freezing up may have saved me. That is only time I've registered a benefit from a Parkinson's symptom. The effect was fleeting.

Over time I have learned that people behave in a rather odd ways if they are driving and they see someone stutter stepping with a walking stick or frozen while trying to take a first step. Even if the person is not on the road or in the crosswalk, they often just stop. The caution is always appreciated, but oftentimes it leads to a "you first, Alfonse" situation. The problem is that the drivers generally want the frozen-in-place person to go ahead, not realizing he or she cannot do that.

As a result, the tension rises for the Parkinson's person who hopes the driver will go ahead and relieve the pressure of going first. The law says drivers must wait for the person to clear the crosswalk but that confounds someone with Parkinson's. This situation is complicated. This cannot be communicated very easily with hand gestures, talking, hoping the driver has good lip reading skills or gestures made with a walking stick. If I can, I back out of the crosswalk or move further away from the road to eliminate the conflict between what traffic laws dictate to drivers and what works for someone with Parkinson's.

On my emergency cartridge trip in this winter situation, the only thing I really could hear was the steady shaking of the plastic bag containing the cause of all this: the printer cartridge. As if on cue, a car now came from my left in the lane I needed to enter next. The communication problem was now a three-way mess. I began to turn back to my car, thinking going home was a capital idea.

Directly behind me I heard a light lilting voice. "I don't think shaking it will fix it." She added, "If I take the bag do you think we can make it into the store?"

"I think so, if somebody doesn't get frustrated and run us over," I replied into the winter wind. Both drivers were being very patient but were noticeably agitated. I could not blame them at all.

As the woman grabbed the bag, I suddenly lost my focus on the cars and the icy wind. I took an extended step which created momentum, making it possible to keep going after a successful first step.

"Hey, wait for me!" the woman yelled. Ice crunched under her boots and car wheels. I kept my head down and plowed forward.

As the automatic door opened to the store, she boxed my shoulder in triumph. No one else in the store knew that this was a grand entrance.

My kind helper took the cartridge to the proper counter, removed her huge coat and asked, "May I help you?" She was easily recognizable as an employee in her colorful red vest. She was the manager or something like that. It is very hard to know these days.

"Winter is not a good time to play in the traffic," she kidded.

"I thought the traffic was playing with me, but I didn't know what the game was," I replied.

She smiled in mutual understanding that no matter what the game was or what the rules were, pedestrians lose.

By the time I bought the new cartridge and a few other items. I was "on." My lady savior gave me a kind of second look and observed, "It looks like you can make it back to the car, right?"

"Yes, no problem," I said.

"I had the guys shovel the crosswalk."

I made it home and printed happily into the night. That's easy because in Montana in the dead of winter night comes at 4:30 p.m.

In addition to the wisdom of always keeping an extra cartridge in my office, this incident taught me something else. We need a massive investment in Parkinson's awareness information available to the general public. This awareness program should encompass many other medical conditions as well. Modern life is so complex that even simple activities can become very difficult to manage and are potentially dangerous in the absence of awareness of people's limits and capacities. Laws do not anticipate all circumstances. As a society we cannot depend on goodhearted people to "save the day" when problems arise. As my wife often says, "Start with good communications and the rest will follow."

SECTION 8: GAINING PERSPECTIVE
I Never Imagined I Would Have a Movement Disorder

Parkinson's changes the place a person occupies in other people's lives. Rarely is this change an improvement. Depending on the person, a specific set of expectations about physical presence comes to be associated with him or her. The way in which people see each other has a lot to do with physical characteristics. The odd thing is that people who may have known each other for 20 or 30 years actually do not see a particular person the same way as others do, much like eyewitness accounts of a crime scene. Each person filters the appearance and presence of a person through their vantage point. This creates a complex grid of perception that affects each person's life in both positive and sometimes negative ways.

Many times a change in a physical condition is accompanied by the need to use an aide such as a walking stick. Its presence in your hands has a very significant effect on people around you. To them it's not an aide, it is a potential source of annoying noise, a tripping hazard or something that reminds them of how authority used sticks to threaten them. So a stick might remind people of a baseball bat in the hands of someone out of control, a rod used to emphasize commands or a stick used to annoy others by an inconsiderate child. It also might cause people to see a person negatively as disabled or in a deteriorating condition, thus automatically limiting the types of interaction with him or her that the person may have actually enjoyed.

This viewpoint can be perceptual or real, and when combined with the practical reality of having to assist another person during an activity, some people withdraw. This reaction is quite different from the attitude toward a person with a temporary injury from which recovery is possible.

One of the truly surprising things about the degenerative characteristics of Parkinson's is that I never imagined myself being disabled. In order to put my disability in perspective I found it useful to remember a person who was extremely courageous in his approach to his movement disorder and to try to draw lessons from that memory. Over 59 years ago when I first met this person with a movement disorder, in this case cerebral palsy, I was 10 years old and never thought that I would have a condition which would cause others to perceive me as disabled. I realize now there was a great and enduring lesson in the way that this person handled himself and his disability that I only hope I can emulate in my management of Parkinson's.

Chapter 24
Looking Back: Lessons from a Dedicated Batboy

When I was about 10 years old, I came across a young man, probably 18, who had cerebral palsy. At the time David was the batboy for the local professional baseball team. That's what impressed me. He moved in a fashion that was unmistakable with his shoulders and arms rising and falling alternately while running bowlegged with his head up and his mouth open. David came at you like a whirlwind. He spoke in a hard-to-understand breathy speech with too much saliva in his mouth. He was constantly slurping to control the fluid. He always wore a baseball cap and was an incredible bundle of energy. The town was small then, and everybody knew him. He taught me a great deal about dignity.

My dad took me to the baseball game one evening, and I saw David down on the field keeping things very lively near the dugout. He was busy stacking bats and getting gloves, catchers' equipment and practice balls set up in their special places. Try as he may to control his actions, he was generating a lot of chaos because of his spontaneous uncontrolled gyrations. He would set up the bats, get it just about done, then his leg would kick out and knock the whole structure down. His ability to handle 10 or 15 baseballs gave calamity a new level of expression. Through his gyrations and shaking it was hard for him to keep a canvas bag right side up or know where the drawstring was located. The shaking would loosen the knot and out would pour balls, spilling into the dugout or rolling toward first base, whereupon he would immediately start a mad chase to corral them.

There were a few of us who were regulars. As I looked around, those who were attending for the first time were all mesmerized watching this somewhat bizarre activity. Everybody else seemed to take no notice at all including the players who just continued about their business dodging and hopping over equipment and occasionally giving a modest assist to David. Amazingly, when the umpire said, "Play ball," everything was in order. David was exhausted. When he held a bat for each player, he could not stop the bat from tapping, thumping the ground or banging on any surface he was near due to his random gyrations. He almost seemed like the secret distraction weapon against the opposing team. You would see batters look him over between pitches. This was subtle. Nothing else about David was.

About the fifth inning one of the local players broke his bat. David exploded into action, grabbing a replacement bat for the player and charging at break neck speed toward home plate.

The umpire jumped to attention, the opposing team catcher hopped out of the way and the local player began to dance like a boxer getting light on his feet as a charging cyclone with a bat came at him. David stopped, held out the bat reducing the gyrations so that the player got it on the third attempt. David then spun around raised his arms in triumph and charged back to his appointed spot. The loudest cheers of the night so far erupted from the stands. The home team seemed to rise to the triumph and went on to win that night.

Later that summer David preformed the same pregame action show described above with very few paying any attention at all. In the seventh inning something very strange occurred. The home team pitcher hit a double, broke his bat, yet managed to slide into second very neatly, surprising the crowd with his athleticism.

The home team was up by one run, and its relief pitchers had demonstrated complete ineffectiveness during this season, leaving a serious lack if anything happened to the pitcher who was now on second base. The manager was hopping around not knowing whether to be happy or mad at the double. But he certainly needed to get a jacket on the pitcher so he didn't get cold and become ineffective. He pointed toward a team jacket and looked at David.

Still holding the broken bat, David grabbed the jacket and bolted toward second base. The silky jacket flew like a Chinese kite above his outstretched arm as the first base coach, the foul line umpire and the first baseman all ran in opposite directions away from him. David was looking up and tripped over first base falling hard on his face sliding through the loose reddish base path dirt. The bat sailed over the second baseman's head. The whole crowd instantly became silent with a collective intake of breath. Everyone near David froze.

David sprung up, shook out the jacket, bowed to the crowd and charged forward, raising his fist in triumph stopping about 10 feet beyond the pitcher on second base. The pitcher walked over and helped David dust off red dirt. David patted him on the back, knocked off his hat, and charged back to his appointed spot, nearly trampling the second baseman on the way.

The crowd went crazy. The second baseman continued to shake. Eventually though, the home team lost because the manager brought in a relief pitcher in the bottom of the eighth inning who gave up two home runs.

After the game, I talked to David who was sporting a new silk jacket presented to him by the pitcher. The pitcher had given it to him as a way to celebrate the only double he ever had. David had made that event much more memorable, even legendary.

When asked by the local radio commentator about David after the game, the manager said, "He keeps us all on our toes and ready to move at any time. Managers like that. No team ever had a more dedicated fan."

David's enthusiasm and ability to find triumph in the disasters yielded by his condition never stood in his way of making sure his team had the bats, balls and anything else they needed to play ball.

SECTION 9:
DISCOVERING DBS
(Deep Brain Stimulation)
SURGERY

I can only describe my eventual decision to have deep brain stimulation (DBS) surgery as a thought experiment, a journey from skepticism to awareness to amazement. It is a way to discover realities beyond experience. We all do it when we try to predict the future or understand something that is beyond our experience. We make educated guesses based on partial information. A person begins by challenging the conventional wisdom that brain surgery is exotic and dangerous.

Was this still true in 2013? This was the question I had to answer. A person can't run an experiment on the effects of his own brain surgery. An individual has no capacity to experience such a procedure, evaluate the results and reverse the experiment. Only a person's imagination may allow someone to project what would happen if an individual determines brain surgery, like DBS, is no longer exotic and dangerous, and may be a viable answer to changing circumstances.

For me, my thought experiment was modest but none-the-less consequential to my future. Sequential decision making provided a path that would work for me. Selecting the sequence was a process of setting priorities.

The first step was setting goals. My first was to maintain a high-quality lifestyle with PD for as long as possible while minimizing the risks of brain surgery. By 2013 my quality of life was declining because of significant increases in dyskinesia caused by the constant increasing dosage of dopamine used to control tremors. I was also in the downward spiral where increased dopamine no longer helped my tremor. Every neurologist and piece of research I could find gave a clear consensus that only DBS could slow down or reverse the downward spiral.

The second goal was to minimize the risks of brain surgery when I deemed DBS was absolutely necessary for my quality of life. The elements of decision-making was straightforward. I gathered as much high-quality information as possible on DBS surgery, including the best location to have it done, the risks, my tolerance for the surgical procedure itself, the post-surgery medical and medication support system, realistic estimates of the probabilities of infection, unanticipated side effects, inherent risks of adverse outcomes, including death, and the effect on my family of each outcome. I had to evaluate each of these questions in the absence of actually doing the surgery and seeing what the consequences were.

Thus, I ran a thought experiment with the intent of maximizing the quality of information. Each of these elements was weighted in the decision to have or not to have DBS surgery. I started with the idea that the possibility of doing it was just as likely as not doing it.

The road I traveled was a rocky twisting journey to DBS surgery. The decision-making process changed my life. I set off down the path when I felt PD had control of its own momentum, and it had begun to dominate my life. My medicine wasn't working as effectively as it had before. As a result, I had to increase the dosage in order to get the same results.

The medicine that was most important to me was the carbidopa/levodopa which was used as a substitute for dopamine. For a very short while, possibly six months, the increases seem to have positive effects. This period gave me the illusion that I could continue to fight and win. That was simply not true. Soon my arms and upper torso were out of control.

It was ultimately a destructive sequence. The more medicine I took for the tremors, which were progressively worse, the more I suffered from the dyskinesia. I had used exercise in the form of handball for the first five years of my Parkinson's development as a way to maintain my body strength, agility, balance and hand eye coordination. When the dyskinesia first started, this approach began to unravel because I could not control my body. I fell a lot. PD-caused freezing was a hazard not only to me but to others around me.

I had already gone to centers of medical excellence to get a second opinion on my treatment, as well as to make sure I was aware of the most current and best practices in managing Parkinson's. This meant visits to Harvard University's teaching hospital — Brigham and Women's Hospital — to meet with researchers in Parkinson's. I had had appointments at University of Southern California Center for Parkinson's and had researched international places of interest such as the University of Zürich using the web. It was with this research that I began to understand the role DBS might play in my future.

Finally, I went to the Mayo Clinic in Rochester, Minnesota for my 10th anniversary evaluation. The neurologist suggested that I was an excellent candidate for DBS surgery. I didn't need to do it immediately, but the neurologist said I should have the surgery before age 74 and carefully monitor my deterioration due to Parkinson's during the next five years or so. This advice was very helpful, in particular regarding the importance of making sure my cognitive abilities remained in place. I was warned their deterioration might make me unqualified for DBS. My local neurologist concurred with this assessment and recommended that I consider DBS in the next year or two.

The DBS procedure was rapidly undergoing technical change and was available in a variety of different institutions. What impressed me was the discovery that this procedure could be done while I was either awake or asleep, depending on the technology available.

Simply put, the DBS procedure involves the insertion of a lead (or probe) with a number of electrodes into the brain into the region of the substantia nigra. The lead is then positioned very carefully in the globus pallidus, thalamus or sub-thalamus. Because the right side of the brain controls the left side of the body and vice versa, two probes are usually inserted.

The probes are then connected by a coated wire extension placed under the skin to a device with a battery pack that controls the signal for two to three years. This device is placed under the chest skin like a pace maker.

At the time the medical community was developing two different procedures. The first, and most frequently used, involved surgery while the patient was awake so that the surgeon could manipulate the placement of the electric probe into a position with the patient's real-time feedback on the most effective position to reducing his or her Parkinson's symptoms.

The second approach was radically different in that the patient was under anesthesia during surgery. Prior to the procedure, the hospital performed an MRI. The images produced were synchronized with a real-time CT scan during surgery to identify the best locations for the probes to reduce symptoms of Parkinson's. The decision to place the leads in a particular place among the possibilities was made by the neurologist and accomplished by the surgeon.

A week later, a second surgery occurred to attach the electronic probes to wires which connect to the control mechanism. The wires were snaked under the skin down to the shoulder, and the control device was placed under the skin on the chest just below the shoulder blade. It was a bit lumpy when completed, but who doesn't have lumps at 67?

Immediately following the second surgery, the neurologist programmed the device, much like a pace maker, to regulate the signal. Then it was time for the patient's brain to adjust to its new instructions.

Once I learned the details of both procedures, it was quite clear to me that I preferred the second approach. The information generated in the first method seemed psychologically very difficult for the patient and might be prone to produce more damage to the brain than the second approach. I discovered that Oregon Health Sciences University, which is only 500 miles from where I lived in Montana, was the pioneer in the second method. Their experts had considerable experience in using it. Their researchers published the findings in peer-reviewed research journals. I also had family and friends in the area to provide support.

Unfortunately, the technology that supports the second procedure is only available in very few places because it is extremely expensive to do so. Not all centers that do DBS surgery have this technology.

In both cases one of the goals of the DBS surgery is the reduction in the amount of levodopa/carbidopa medicine a person has to take. The procedures are designed to reduce tremors and other aspects of Parkinson's. A second goal is to maximize the time the procedure is effective, which might be 10 years or more depending on the situation.

Before being approved to do the DBS surgery the patient must undergo an exhaustive set of psychological and physical tests given by the neuropsychologist and neurologist. Somewhat to my surprise, the neuropsychology aspect is very important. The patient must be cognitively intact and capable psychologically of dealing with brain surgery and the impact of DBS on his or her emotional state. In addition, the progression of PD must not be so severe that a patient cannot expect reduction of tremors and other PD symptoms. Therefore, this is a judgment call on the patient's part and on the part of the neurologist and neuropsychologist as to whether or not someone with PD stands to gain substantially from the procedure.

There is a risk in waiting too long. A person's

deterioration may disqualify them either psychologically, physically or by some combination of both. In my case I was qualified on both criteria. When I made the decision to go ahead I was 67 years old, in good health, physically strong in the sense that I exercised a great deal and was fit, having lost 50 pounds over the past four years or so and maintained that weight for some time (6 feet, 2 inches tall and 200 pounds). I'm sure that every situation varies considerably, but that was my situation at the time.

This decision process took me approximately five years. Fortunately, I did not wait too long. Also, I did not do it too early. I decided to wait approximately two years beyond my Mayo Clinic neurologist's recommendation. This also was a time when the method involving the patient being asleep was refined, and the research published.

It's brain surgery. No matter what, it is serious. The risks are significant if anything goes wrong. The probabilities are very low of a stroke or infection, but the decision must be considered carefully.

I went from skepticism to awareness to amazement about the procedure over that five-year period. Skepticism involved the evaluation of the risk verses promised outcomes. Awareness came as a result of two things: first the realization that my medicine no longer worked effectively and caused dyskinesia that I could not tolerate and still live my life. Second, I thoroughly researched and understood the procedures available to me and chose not only which procedure, but where it would be done. Amazement came with the realization that my tremor was gone, the dyskinesia was gone and many of my symptoms had abated.

The remaining problem was and remains a loss of balance at times and problems initiating walking. These are continuing issues. The neurologist was very clear that DBS does not promise improved balance. Balance issues can be mitigated by a commitment to physical therapy and retraining of brain pathways controlling walking and movement. This commitment to physical therapy is within my power to accomplish, and I realize that I am fighting a battle against the progressive deterioration inherent in PD. I know that the DBS has not cured my Parkinson's, but it has relieved me from some of the symptoms and from the problem with medication side effects for at least a period of time. The respite maybe 10 years, maybe five years, but at least I have had some substantial improvement.

How does a person view their own brain? I've always felt mine was a "happening place," where reality emerges on a fantastic screen. Thoughts of the nature of my brain grew more significant to me as I contemplated brain surgery.

When person begins planning for someone to intrude into his brain, the ebbs and flows of the 24-hour news cycle seem unimportant. Instead, he starts thinking about the very nature of brain surgery. First, there is the barbarity of having most of your head shaved, your skull drilled like a two-fingered bowling ball and wires inserted from cortex through cerebellum to what some describe as "that reptilian part" at the base of the brain, allowing a device to fire electrical current through the synapses. I couldn't help but be amazed that medical science has reached a point where a surgeon and a team of mysteriously dressed acolytes could enter my cranium like good campers, pack it in and pack it out, and leave no trace of their presence except fine wires that allowed me to recover lost capacities. With remote imaging combining the MRI and real-time CT scan imagery so precise that no blood is released, the ancient part of my brain is connected to the marvels of modern science. It's like Tarzan finally communicating with the chimp.

My thought process randomly switched from one view to the other as the date of the surgery loomed larger on the horizon. One of the interesting and perplexing problems facing those who have had DBS brain surgery is that, until recently, there was no reasonable explanation as to why it worked. It's called DBS, which could stand for "Definitely

Big Scam," or it could stand for deep brain stimulation, which sounds either frightening or New Age.

To the best of my understanding what actually happens is a lot like the way sound-canceling earphones deal with the problem of separating the signal from ambient noise for the listener, only in this case DBS provides clarity for those centers in the brain that control movement. The electrical stimulus cancels the noise produced by Parkinson's, leaving the brain more capable of discerning the correct signal. This concept is something abstract to most of us, but the various potential meanings of the concept have been made eminently clear by Nate Silver in his brilliant book "The Signal and the Noise." He clarifies ways to find the essential information in the barrage of stimuli we are bombarded with daily. With no way to sort the information we are overwhelmed much like a PD sufferer is in the frozen state of Parkinson's. DBS allows one's brain to find the signal.

So how does one bridge between the gap between the barbaric and the amazing state of medical science? There's a visceral response to the very idea of brain surgery among most of those contemplating it. Rational friends and family members typically say, "It's your decision ... I'll back you up." But ultimately you must make the choice. It's a scary one.

I made up my mind after carefully weighing the risks and rewards systematically, primarily because I could have the procedure done while I was asleep. My fear in doing surgery while I was awake was that my reading of the improvement in my in symptoms would not be reliable with two holes drilled in my head and my skull rigidly anchored to an operating table with bolts. The second reason I made my decision is the improvement in precision that has been achieved with virtual imagery. The old practice of "fishing around" for the right spot has been replaced with the precise placement via three-dimensional imaging. I was ready to go with virtual imagery and three-dimensional coordinates knowing the surgeon and the technology were in synch rather than depending on the decision I would make while I fought the urge to flee the operating room as quickly as possible.

The clincher was that Parkinson's is a progressive disease, and mine had progressed to the point where more meds caused me more trouble and fewer meds caused me more trouble. There was nowhere to go for relief except DBS.

Luckily, medical science had radically progressed in just a few years. How had it happened? There was a marvelous blend of private initiative and public commitment to research, leading to the modern medical practices that have replaced barbaric drilling of holes in skulls and bloodletting that represented best practice over the last few thousand years. Modern medical science is not perfect but the improvement is profound. When a procedure, such as DBS, has been proven clinically, the amazing people in the health care system provide a path to a better life. Once you've made the decision, it is amazing how many of those close to you rally round your decision to take the risk.

It is an easy choice when you hear the sounds of grandchildren screeching with joy as they plunge head first down a 15-foot water slide to see who can make the biggest splash. You must be ready to join them for as long as you can, accepting the fact that life sometimes involves taking risks to reap the rewards life offers.

Chapter 25
Brain Surgery

While immersed in a fog of anesthesia, I was concerned I might awake from my brain surgery looking a little like Frankenstein, perhaps scaring small children and whole villages. After all, they had drilled two holes into my skull to insert wires with anchors that could resemble horns. Instead, I was greeted by smiling family and friends who calmed my fears, and I began the recovery process fairly perky. I knew in advance that I would have two electrodes inserted in my brain with some sort of device holding each one in place. Fortunately they are fairly flat as opposed to the horns that were used some years back, so I avoided the old fashioned protruding plugs that looked as though they could be attached to jumper cables. If you look at the stitches on my bald head, someone might observe that I was I was kicked in the head by a small donkey.

The first surgery seemed to be a success in the eyes of my family. My wife, my daughter and her husband, as well as the four grandchildren, came to Portland to support me. My wife was extraordinarily calm while keeping fear and hope in balance. She sported a "the show must go on" attitude with realistic expectations. She knew the surgery was technically successful, and that a positive attitude was crucial in these situations. You could see her resolve.

My daughter had put together a blog called "Den's brain blog" to keep all our friends updated on my status. The thousand plus hits it received were wonderfully supportive, and I recommend this kind of communication to anyone in my situation.

My son-in-law had brought the grandchildren along because he had an instinct that family learning came from actual life experience. He has an "I've got your back, no problem" attitude.

The grandchildren were amazing. Perfect for their ages ranging from four to 12. The four-year-old girl had worked on a whole routine of cute that would make Shirley Temple update her script. She charmed me.

The seven-year-old boy described in detail his version of the surgery, and how I came to look "wacky."

The 10-year-old girl gave me tender hugs and the sense that the kind of confidence that she brought to her gymnastics was the therapy I needed. I was ready to team up, but no balance beam. I immediately felt stronger.

The eldest, a 12-year-old girl, an artist at heart, stood toward the back of the room. I could see her quiver under her perfect straw hat with a blue bow and simple beautiful summer dress, nearly tearing, but smiling so broadly that she glowed. She came over and gave me a tender kiss as I said, "I'll be okay."

"I know, but it's still scary." She knew enough to see danger but flew on the wings of the miracle. Like my daughter and her mother before her, my granddaughter was developing the capacity to take reality and find the part that carries inspiration and not just the challenge of the day. I was thrilled.

Inspired, strengthened, charmed, protected, not overwhelmed and with the love and strength of my life partner I emerged from the fog ready for the next phase:

recovery.

I had also thought carefully about what was coming. The miracle begins with the people who created the technology and imagined a better way to do this procedure. They imagined doing the procedure while the patient was asleep, an amazing progression in the process. Secondly, they created a mechanism where the precision of placement of the electronic probes could be virtually exact. Finally, they lowered the probabilities of infection and bleeding as well as stroke. These are not discrete or mutually exclusive goals. Pursuing them all at once improves each. The technology developed is extraordinarily refined. I don't presume to know how it all works but as I rolled into the operating room I was overwhelmed by the number of people there for this event and the interactive complexity of the systems. Crucial to this process is something called CereTom, a device that allows real-time CT scan imagery to be integrated with an MRI, creating a three-dimensional virtual GPS location target while facilitating insertion of the electronic device in one attempt. To be able to sleep through this was a blessing, and I raise a toast of good Irish whiskey to all those who preceded me in this procedure who were awake. I pay homage to their courage and fortitude.

My friends backed me in many ways by supporting my wife and family by simply "being there virtually" on the day of the surgery. I remember vividly a stalwart friend visiting me in the fog of recovery looking about in amazement at the technological apparatus monitoring my existence. He was there through the fog, and that counts. I believe, for example, if you speak the name of someone you care for, they reappear for a moment. I believe that positive thoughts are cumulative, and their force can challenge negative outcomes for dominance. No guarantees, but possibilities can be imagined that outnumber a limited range of outcomes.

The real challenge arises when you have to deal with the

unintended consequences of all this technology. When you are so closely monitored, chaos can erupt. There should be a way to notify the attending nurse and/or a backup when your blood pressure rises, heart rate falls, the IV comes out, or you shift in bed without alarming the entire ICU. The problem, of course, is lost sleep. Sleep is very likely a major component of the healing process. This is a problem that appears to be universal in hospitals around the country.

If you think immigration brings us only the unskilled and trouble makers and is a bad thing, you have not been in an urban hospital lately. Nursing care is an international phenomenon, and the dedication of the multinational staff at health care facilities is outstanding.

If you think that there is a way to find the perfect economy by relying solely on the private sector or the public sector I also suggest that you do not get sick. It is obvious when you are in the bowels of the hospital where the public and private sector work together to provide the research and resources to make DBS "brain surgery" possible. My friend was observing the remarkable technology resulting from the partnership. This technology is specific enough to keep me alive and general enough to save lives in dire emergencies. Sometimes clarity comes not from imaginary experience but from the real thing.

The learning curve is high and steep in hospitals. It is overcome by the merging of data in modern hospitals. I wound up in the hospital an additional day because of negative response to anesthesia. By the second surgery to attach the probes to wires and the control mechanism, the staff had worked through the problem and found a solution. I certainly never felt like a number but a living breathing patient.

Today this second surgery is completed so efficiently that it is an outpatient procedure. There are no unexplained lumps so the surgeons must have packed out what they packed in, leaving only what they intended.

My nephew, Robert, came from Texas to help me and his aunt deal with the second surgery and the trip home. He began working on my golf grip as he wheeled me around town. He was just what I needed, someone who was looking past the present, pointing toward the future and dealing with the fact that I had nearly lost my grip.

As we flew back to Montana, I was able to note how many people whom I had never met who took time out from their lives to pass positive thoughts my way. Every good thought counts.

Chapter 26
Doing the DBS

The third stage of DBS is the turning on of the electrodes implanted in the brain and the control devise implanted in my chest. This is where reality either bites or a path to a better tomorrow emerges.

The neurologists wait roughly a month after the surgery to make sure there's no rejection of the devices or infections before they actually turn the controller on. I'm not sure at that point whether I became a cyborg or just bionic, but I'm definitely better off.

When it was finally time to "juice up" the DBS system, the step was the final culmination of a series of decisions I'd made. Once the electrodes were implanted in my brain, I was committed. Now I was playing poker with no wild cards and betting heavily on an inside straight in a room with expert players.

It turned out that the players were all on my side. How I reacted to the DBS determined how much I got out of it. I must let it work, not fight for control. I must play my best hand and not depend on the inside straight. Giving up control was the hardest part so far.

So what does the DBS controller do?

A neurologist, physician's assistant, a representative of the company that manufactured the device, a significant other or the patient can operate a programming device that connects with the controller that had been implanted in the chest. (More details on that later.) At the extreme the operator can turn the device off or on. These are the facts.

I once thought that "just the facts" would lead us to a unique conclusion. That is not true.

The first thing I did when looking the neurologist in the eye was to be get him to agree (no reluctance on his part) that I had started the artistic part of the process. Programming the device began a three-month long, three-step process of adjusting the signals to the brain, reviewing the response and "tweaking" the parameters of the device after that.

"Juicing." "Tweaking." Do we use these terms to soften the reality of what is going on? We are altering the signals the brain relies on to function! Isn't that serious business? Oh well, it is just, "messing" with the brain, right?

I must admit that my first concern was the hope that all the wireless devices in the clinic were on a different frequency from my device. If you get interference, would it be like a small airplane crashing? The neurologist assured me that interference would not happen. I wondered if he knew how many cell phones there were in a hospital populated by a plethora of 25-year-olds. I was just nervous.

The first "juicing" is a leap into the unknown. What I experienced might have been a unique experience. In fact, words are a poor device to explain what the feeling was like. I can only describe it as a stunning realization of how phenomenal and complex the brain is. Frankly, we should be much more careful when considering playing football, taking a header in soccer, boxing, or not wearing a helmet while bicycling, etc. I have done each and "lucky" ought to be my nickname or maybe that's why I am engaged in this endeavor. I will never know.

Miracles are not always easy to understand or to comprehend. Miracles are something I haven't experienced before. There is no learning curve for a unique event. What I can assure you is that this experience was mind altering. It was not terrifying. You only get to this point in the process after being carefully screened for mental stability.

The process is a multifaceted probing of the different impacts, frequency and signal strength have on the behavioral aspects of your Parkinson's. From tremor to gait to vision and speech to cognitive powers and autonomic functions, such as breathing, the limits are tested and settings are determined by trial and error. When limits were reached, there was no doubt in my mind that those were the limits. Tremors can be ramped up or down, speech can be slurred or not, vision can be rendered clear or become triple, the ability to walk or move one's limbs can be frozen or free and, of course, this is the rub; there are trade-offs. It's like economics, nothing is free. At one setting I simply folded up like a robot who suddenly lost power. It was frightening but not terrifying.

Speech, clarity of vision, tremor, and mobility, gait, cognitive powers are not set independently; they are jointly determined. For example if you have five behavioral goals and two of them are essential, such as vision and tremor control, and must be set at a specific levels to be tolerable, then one has three choices among the other goals, all of which must not interfere with the vision or tremor control settings. For example, speech and mobility must be set at levels that are suboptimal given their rate of trade-off and the absolute constraints necessary to achieve the goals of vision clarity and tremor control. Reality bites. As the search proceeded, I felt the trade-offs. The electric adjustments became art as well as science.

We can choose our settings and be a different person each time to the world. Likewise many different versions of me are possible. But in each case, the range must be within my tolerances. Not all are perfect, such as bit of slurred speech to achieve mobility, but all are variations of what is possible.

Among the seven or eight billion of us there could be nearly an infinite variety of settings. There were nearly an infinite set of lighting conditions as Monet panted the Rouen cathedral in the changing light of the day, but only a few were impressions that were distinctly different. Only thirty were painted. We each are like the cathedral. We are unique, but leave many different impressions depending on who is observing and what we are engaged in at the time. Our DNA allows only so many variations to be human among the choices of various combinations of vision, speech, mobility, cognitive powers and autonomic functions open to the neurologist.

Cogito ergo sum is not just a Latin saying. I am human because I think. The process of searching the brain for the DBS settings which allow a person to appear human is testing those limits to find a set of attributes with which we each can live. The fact that we can do this is amazing. The result is a miracle of imagination and technology. We have gone from drilling holes in the skull to relieve pressure to precisely controlling our vision or to controlling the way we walk or whether we have tremors. Someone might say we can change the soul as perceived by others.

That raises questions that are cosmic and philosophical. That's a bridge too far. I no longer have the shakes; I do not move uncontrollably; I can walk; my speech is not slurred. But I have fuzzy vision sometimes, and I still take a great deal of medicine and fall when I am forced to move quickly. I have balance issues. I still have Parkinson's. It inevitably will erode my gains. Yet I have maybe ten years or more to love my wife, enjoy my family and see the precious next generation come of age. In addition, I have the chance to enjoy the company of friends. My decision to have DBS was a risk worth taking.

SECTION 10: CONTINUING ON

After DBS, life just continued on. I quickly realize that PD was still a major component of my life. In my case the adjustment to DBS and the new lower dosages of meds took approximately one year. I had expected the adjustment to new levels of medication to take about six months. As a result, the mismatch of expectations and reality had to be reconciled, not only for myself, but for those around me. One of the most difficult aspects of DBS is that friends, family and acquaintances have expectations that are all over the map.

Once I had the surgery, the most common comment with which I was greeted with was, "You look great." In the beginning, I replied, "Thanks." That pretty much ended the conversation. I learned a more engaging response was, "I am still able to play golf," or "I can still fly fish with my nephew."

In the movie "Papillion" Steve McQueen is in solitary, and when food is served, he asks his trusted neighbor, "How do I look?" The response was always, "Fine."

The question was not helpful. "Do I look strong enough to escape?" would have netted the answer McQueen was actually looking to receive — either yes or no.

In my case the reference to golf or fishing changes the focus from "looks" to "behavior," and it opens the conversation rather than stops it. Any attempt to explain an answer different from "thanks" without control of the context is often boring, lengthy and imprecise. I do not want to be that boring person who always talks about PD, DBS and my health.

The approach I took to avoid that fate was to live my life as close as I could to its past history and get on with adapting my behavior given the impact of DBS. In this way the community around me adjusted to what people could observe, rather than hearing me talk about what I could do in the abstract.

Chapter 27
"Survivor"

The idea of a day trip on a 40-foot catamaran off Tobago (the smaller island of Trinidad and Tobago (TT)) doesn't sound like a scary proposition, even when you have Parkinson's. My wife's often repeated mantra, "You should do something scary every year just to prove you're alive," usually comes as some advance notice of an upcoming event, such as "We're going zip-lining in Costa Rica, or "We are going back country mountain biking in Montana," but this adventure was a complete surprise, even to her.

It all began with a somewhat unnerving drive through the narrow roads and spooky traffic on Tobago. Driving on the island is a continuous game of "chicken," with uninsured and inexperienced drivers careening around blind corners. They drive with an urgency that would make an ambulance seem to be standing still while on the way to a victim in cardiac arrest. That combined with the fact that it's all done according to British rules of the road makes an American like me find closing one's eyes to be really a good idea.

Grateful, we arrived unscathed at the designated bar identified as "the place to pick up the boat." It became immediately apparent that this wasn't a walk down a marina dock to step on a gentle gangplank and into the boat. Once we negotiated a garishly multicolored dance bar and dodged the 6-foot 3-inch proprietress towering in 6-inch stiletto heels who announced we must pay to pee (five TT dollars) unless we bought a beer for 20 TT dollar, we passed through a gauntlet of coconut milk hawking, machete wielding, unemployed young men to get to the beach.

Successful negotiation of this ambush brought me to shore's edge where I could see my goal: an 8-foot Zodiac careening back and forth in the surf. This was to be our transportation to the distant catamaran which, at first glance, seemed extremely small until I realized it was quite a ways offshore.

I was greeted in a most friendly fashion by a very fit, smiling man who gave me a German-accented hello using Trinidadian English. He was still working on this second language after 13 years on the island. Once the greetings were exchanged, apparently to him it was time to "hop" into the Zodiac between waves despite my cane and obvious Parkinson's freeze.

Suddenly, the captain became cognizant of my mobility problems and took my cane to make sure I didn't stab the Zodiac in an effort to get in. Somehow I was going to have to roll up my long pants and wade out beyond the most severe crashing waves in order to "leap" in the boat. This would be reasonably easy in normal circumstances except I am not normal. I have balance problems. I was now required to wade without a cane, in spite of the fact my legs were "frozen" to the sand beneath my feet.

There were two things in my favor: First, the Zodiac had a low profile, not presenting too much of an obstacle. Second, I'd grown used to timing things. With supreme concentration and a massive dose of adrenaline topping off my dopamine, I managed to step into the rising and falling boat, turn and sit down. To those watching me navigate into the inflatable boat, which was approximately the same size as my body, the possibility of capsizing was a real concern since my movement placed the center of gravity three feet above the water line.

This problem was solved by having my wife get in on the other side while the captain leapt over the outboard motor turning it on in midair. We motored out to the catamaran.

With a radiant smile the captain said, "Velcome, no dramas, don't worry, getting on the boat will be a piece of cake. My crew vill help you vith getting on the catamaran."

"I hope they are strong," I replied.

Silence.

Though remaining confused by the mixture of Caribbean and German accents, I was pleased to be moving. No longer fearing we were capsizing, we moved toward the catamaran which was proudly named Picante. I was puzzled by the choice of name since picante was normally used for the temperature of hot sauce, not German boats. I stopped concentrating on language issues because I spotted the "crew."

Waiting on the catamaran was a very small, native island woman wearing only a scant brilliant white bikini. She was busy tying down halyards and other sailing stuff in preparation for our departure. No one else appeared. As we pulled in behind the catamaran, the captain announced "no problems" and directed my wife to get off first.

I am 6 feet 1 inch tall and 220 pounds while the only "crew" was busy limbering up, stretching to 5 feet tall, while barely weighing in at 100 pounds by my quick calculation. The back of the boat was at least eight feet above the water with no apparent handholds to help someone climb on.

I immediately began seeing myself going back to shore and reversing the Zodiac entry process. However, the captain and the one-woman crew assured me that all was well, and I decided in a moment of delirium to believe them.

My wife nimbly scaled the obstacle called the fantail and prepared to watch the goings-on while encouraging me to get aboard. Suddenly, the "crew," the bikini-clad tiny woman, grabbed me under the arms in a hold designed to get me seated on the catamaran while my feet were still in the Zodiac.

The old saying about being "between the devil and the deep blue sea" came to mind as the Zodiac rose and fell with the wave action in exact opposition to the catamaran's movements. In one motion she spun me around so my feet were on the catamaran.

"Stand up, I've got you," she said.

As I tried to comply, the mostly naked crewmember dropped-down around my waist and said, "Push off on my thigh." Grabbing her thigh with enough force to turn it white at the pressure point, I was suddenly upright.

"Good job," my wife said.

"Don't you go lean'n overboard," the "crew" said. She was still wrapped around my waist while balancing against the side wall of the fantail. I have yet to figure out how she managed this contortion. At this point the captain announced that he was going back for the other guests and promptly took off in the Zodiac. I recognized that he thought I was on the boat while I thought I was about halfway home.

The rest of the ascent seemed possible. With a little push here and a nudge there, I was in the cockpit and able to get a seat on my own. It was then that I met the crew face-to-face after already having been involved with the "crew" back to belly. She was delightful. When I asked her name she gleefully replied "Minelist," an occult name her mother found somewhere meaning "survivor." She had numerous scars on her face that made me think of those one would see in Africa, sort of beauty marks among tribal people. The scars did not detract but rather enhanced the impression that she was fierce and strong beyond her diminutive stature. I needed no convincing.

At that point the rest of the "sailors for the day" had arrived and all agreed that it was amazing that I was able to get up on the boat. I observed that I had been involved, but that Minelist had done the lion's share of the work and lifting. They heard what I said, but didn't really take it literally.

However, a couple of hours later, after sailing through a torrential squall into beautiful sunshine with the ocean turning from angry gray to Caribbean azure blue, they saw I wasn't just being over complementary. The "crew" managed during this time to charm everyone, prepare a magical luncheon with a Tobago spiced flavor that was the quality of any I have had ever tasted and zipped effortlessly around the boat seeming to always anticipating the captain's directions.

Several passengers commented on her abilities to the captain. "When she's not here saving my bacon, she's off fishing expertly in these very dangerous waters," he responded.

"I love my life," the "crew" announced. Her point of view was contagious, and soon everyone on board the catamaran seemed to be an extension of her personal enthusiasm. The smile on the captain's face and her warming return smile made several of us feel the captain and the crew were "involved." I think the captain sensed this and cut off the rush to judgment by saying, "You might know my wife. She's with Crown Point."

Slightly embarrassed, "Oh yes, I know her" responses from the local guests followed. At this point the snorkelers had snorkeled and the sunbathers were fried, the jib had flown, and we were peacefully cruising our way back to the original mooring.

As it was the captain's custom to deal with a potential problem before anything else, I was to be first to disembark, this time with the entire audience of "day sailors" on the catamaran for an up close observation of my dissent back to the Zodiac. I honestly thought the 8-foot drop would be more daunting than the 8-foot ascent. To some extent that was true, but the word "drop" hardly describes the exotic manipulation of me that ensued. The "crew," still in her tiny white bikini, announced that I was to grab a halyard, then I was to step off the fantail into what appeared to me to be an empty void with no step within four feet of my foot.

"I've got you mon, don't lean too far out," she stated.

There was no chance I was going to lean too far out. What happened next from my point of view was that this incredible woman merged with me in such a fashion where I felt there was no separation. Suddenly, I had two additional arms and legs emerging from my back as though I had become an Irish version of the Hindu God Vishnu.

I must have made a noise that sounded somewhat erotic as I caught my breath.

"I've got to move my leg over you now," she said while I was being floated down to the step.

The combination of sound and action made the audience of "sailors" utter observations such as "Interesting," "How's that feel?" and "Who's doing what to whom?" A salacious request from a male friend volunteered, "I'm next."

To my perception, I seemed to float in the air, able to reach the step while regaining my consciousness of the pitching of the Zodiac below me. The weakness in my knees and stiffness that accompanies my Parkinson's would normally make this movement impossible. The "crew" seemed to anticipate this reality for me as she had anticipated the captain's needs. From behind me she said, "I've got you. Just slide down me and relax."

From the "sailors" there were collective, individual and breathy observations that all seem to express the sense captured by the question, "She said what?"

I slid down her safely, but gingerly, to the Zodiac.

"There you go, mon," the "crew" said.

"Velcome," the captain said, speaking as though there was nothing remarkable about my experience.

My wife joined me on the top-heavy Zodiac for the trip to shore. I again felt "involved" in my exit from the catamaran, and I have a continuing sense that the "crew" was "committed" in the sense that a she took all the risk to life and limb, and I received the rewards.

My dear friends and family, who constituted the sailors that day, all observed that the "crew" had seemingly cast a spell on the moment and managed to effortlessly do what seemed impossible objectively when you compared the two of us physically. On the beach, I declared it was time for a "dark and stormy," a drink of dark rum, ginger ale and fresh limes well-known in the Caribbean. It was definitely appropriate.

Chapter 28
Looking Ahead

As I think of ways to conclude this book, it is my observation that it really can't end or reach a conclusion. My nephew Robert from Texas made the same observation, confirming my gut feeling. I regard this as an interim report on what I've discovered so far.

Once you realize that the situation is permanent and that Parkinson's is forever a part of your life, you can choose to adapt to the ever-changing symptoms or you can give up and let it overwhelm your life. Making this choice has significant implications for others as well as yourself. I have given an example of how fiercely and dedicatedly someone with cerebral palsy faced life by finding something he loved and committing to making it happen for others. I'm sure he knew that he was a unique part of the baseball game. Rather than interpret the crowd's reaction as negative, he chose to regard it as triumphant, winning over even the most cynical people in the stands.

I feel somewhat the same. As with all theater, there are elements of comedy and tragedy in every great performance. Shakespeare observed in "As You Like It," that, "All the world's a stage, and all the men and women merely players:

they have their exits and their entrances; and one man in his time plays many parts …"

When someone is diagnosed with Parkinson's, early-onset or in their 60s, a person must come to terms with the fact that it's going to be forever present. The ability to process this reality, that a condition is forever, is something that I have observed in numerous examples of courageous people over my 70 years.

A compelling example is the case of a young woman that I have known since she was a child. Affectionately known as "Edie," she was born with dwarfism into the most supportive family one can imagine. The family created a space where she was normal and treated as such in all respects. This environment allowed her to chart her own path without being suffocated by others' definition. In this marvelously constructed, but bounded environment, she thrived.

As she matured, I skied with her down the face of Whitefish Mountain, an activity that is best described as chasing a snowball. We teamed up as tennis partners for a family tournament, the odd couple, with my 6-foot 2-inch height dominating her 3-foot 5-inch body. She served with pinpoint accuracy and volleyed ferociously while I played the net and scrambled for the lob shots. We lost in the finals to a team that included a three-time state champion and a skilled veteran of numerous regional tournaments. While Edie was in college she was my partner in a snorkeling adventure off Isla de Vieques. She took on the challenge and was fearless and curious. Since then she's become a wife, mother, statistician and cancer survivor, carrying on fearlessly in the face of daunting challenges.

Edie has been an inspiration to all who have lifelong challenges they must face in the lonely place where courage lives so they can reconstruct their future. As a point of reference, she is a great reminder of overcoming ever-changing challenges.

As with most people facing a slowly emerging condition such as PD, I knew what to do intellectually before beginning to train myself in my new reality. By keeping the focus on self-control and consistent behavior while working diligently but carefully, I was able to acquire appropriate responses to Parkinson's through learning by trial and error. In normal circumstances many skills, resources and bits of wisdom we have learned in the past lay dormant, but resurface when needed to provide us with the means to problem solve any situation.

Being unprepared for Parkinson's demands before having it is the natural state of affairs. This does not mean people are naturally complacent; it simply means that Parkinson's hits like a slow-motion car wreck out of nowhere. That does not mean that we have no inherent strategies to cope with PD. We have the means to invent ourselves again and then to repeat the process, continually accommodating the challenges of the future. Parkinson's is just one of the issues, among others such as aging, retirement, the coming-of-age of our children, death of our parents and all those rites of passage of our lives that must be confronted as we move through time.

Someday, we may have predictors, genetically based and/or environmentally determined, that will warn us when Parkinson's will present itself. But that is not the case now. Parkinson's develops along a pathway that cannot be controlled. And people dealing with it must train themselves to respond to its impact on life. This means acquiring information to make informed choices and keeping up with an ever-changing situation.

In the case of Parkinson's, it is important to rely on finding the right fit among choices in the medical services community, disciplined use of medicine, rigorous exercise, the right diet, the appropriate attitude and self-discipline to guide the choice between action and rest, knowledge of when to depend on other people and the ability to employ general skills learned through life experiences.

Most of all, Parkinson's requires flexibility and recognition that constant change is necessary as symptoms progress. In fact, dealing with the disease's constant permutations is one of the most difficult challenges. At the point of diagnosis, no choices exist beyond going along for the ride while, at the same time, figuring out ways to cope and hold on tight so that Parkinson's does not destroy life's remaining possibilities.

The idea of managing Parkinson's disease is much more realistic than any pretense that controlling it is possible. The only controls to be developed are self-controls. Few people ever come to a stalemate with Parkinson's. It will never stop nor yield to any force or subterfuge.

My assessment builds on years of dealing with the consequences that unfold as my reality changes. Parkinson's changes life by altering just about everything. Slowly at first and then faster and faster, Parkinson's redirects energies. Whatever may have been a person's place in society before Parkinson's, it will change as the disease continues to progress.

Parkinson's is a process of inevitable sustained decline and increase in the power of the symptoms to disrupt and diminish a person's ability to control physical, behavioral and even mental capabilities. This is a reality. As a result people with Parkinson's must continue to adjust to the changing demands of the condition.

A person with Parkinson's must transform into a master of damage control management to combat the disease which will continually attack the body and personality over time. To undergo this type of transformation requires communication with others. Building a community that can accept this type of personal transformation is important to a person going through each stage.

What I have found necessary to deal with Parkinson's disease is to assume a positive, even good-humored, attitude and, at times, a cold-blooded posture toward Parkinson's. A realistic attitude allows the ability to set goals which are linked to meaningful actions. Our success in containing neurological degenerative conditions such as Parkinson's is measured in our ability to retain dignity, opportunity, self-respect, reputation, membership in our community and participation in family activities over the course of the progression of the disease. People will certainly have to consider professional help from others such as clinical psychologists, health professionals, social workers and counselors to help them deal with issues as they present themselves. The professionals can instruct. However, they depend on the individual to take action on their own. Life will be 1 percent instruction and 99 percent homework. It will be tiring and unrelenting. The benefit is maintaining quality of life as long as possible and having a life worth living. Not a bad trade off.

Maintaining a positive attitude is accomplished by sharing confidences with friends and family, working with a medical care team and accepting the help of a stranger gracefully. Psychologists are accurate when they emphasize the importance of anticipating the future by controlling daydreams, self-imagery and rehearsal of possible scenarios so that experiences are self-affirming rather than self-defeating. In the activities of day-to-day life, how a person imagines reality defines how a person greets the world.

Many of the problems that emerge in dealing with the symptoms of PD offer a curious opportunity to test the limits of our creative side. For example, taking on new challenges and redefining your role in your peer group may offer new perspectives for each individual in the group.

There is no doubt that Parkinson's will ultimately restrict a person's life. This fact could lead to pessimism. But restrictive limits ignore the magical property built into the structure of the universe: every time something infinite is made smaller what remains still has an infinite number of possibilities. This strange fact leads to optimism if one looks carefully at the new set of possibilities that emerge from any situation. The choice between optimism and pessimism is up to the individual. Optimism stems from confidence and an experimental attitude toward the world as the person's world changes.

The message here is not simply *carpe diem* but "bring it on." The Irish seem to have a saying for nearly everything. "May the road rise to meet you" only has meaning as long as you're on the road. A warrior bushwhacks his or her way around the path Parkinson's presents. The future is full of stories as yet untold. We must be determined, ready to handle uncertainty.

It is essential to take on the unknown, acknowledge what cannot be managed and target all efforts at the rest.

The opportunity exists to pass on what one has been learned to someone else. Having benefited from those who make sure we are not isolated, it is important to reciprocate by making sure others are not left alone either.

Telling my story, as we all should, is accomplished by communicating with as many people as I can reach with this book. When we touch other lives by sharing our stories of triumph and struggle and learning through trial and error, we are never outnumbered or alone.

EPILOGUE: OUT OF THE BLUE

Over the course of the last three years while writing this book, I have experienced more of the unsettling effects of the wild thing (a change in the effectiveness of my medications) which I now regard as par for the course. The fact that I have ever evolving Parkinson's and take medication that has fixed medicinal properties means I have to be very aware of my mind and body at all times. This reality is an ever present property of the off-kilter relationship between Parkinson's and medicine.

One of my medications has become addictive and less effective. This means that I need to stop taking it and find a reasonable substitute. At first I thought this could be done in a fairly short period of time, such as a week. I was seriously wrong.

As previously mentioned, I'm viewing this book as an interim report on my experience with Parkinson's and how it plays out as I interact with the rest of the world. As an example of continuing acts of the kindness of others, I had another in a series of thoughtful and surprising occurrences happen for my benefit. On a recent Saturday, I was arriving at the Missoula airport on a trip that originated from Lugano, Switzerland.

I was deplaning in a wheelchair because the flight time that day had made my legs so stiff I barely could walk. At the door of the plane, I was met by a gate agent with a wheelchair. I asked to immediately be taken to the bathroom. The gate agent took me up the gateway and realized on the way that she could not leave the gate door unattended and could not take me where I needed to go. My wife had been separated from me due to confusing signals in the general chaos of the plane's arrival. She had my cane. I could not wait and began to stumble toward the restroom without my cane. The gate agent was in a hopeless situation given her assigned duties; most importantly she could not leave the gate unattended because of security issues.

Out of nowhere Scott emerged from among the departing passengers. He'd overheard us and recognized the difficulty of the situation, He grabbed the wheelchair, brought it to me and solved the problem. I had barely a chance to thank him before he had to join his departure queue. I'm surprised I didn't hear the roar of a Harley over the noise of the lounge.

These types of experiences, which I have shared with you throughout this book, have happened to me on many occasions over the course of my Parkinson's journey. The purpose of this book is to encourage those who have Parkinson's to venture into the world, not to simply accept a life with Parkinson's but to "take it on."

There are a large number of thoughtful, observant people who will step in when needed to assist in a predicament. The world appears busy, somewhat self-centered and chaotic. Evan so, there is inevitably someone who is ready to help, who comes forward to save the day. Scott is just the latest in my experience.

Before Parkinson's put me on the journey it dictated some 16 years ago, I was like most people who hardly noticed the acts of discrete assistance that went on around me. I always helped when I could. I just never saw the whole picture. I still am astonished at the good that lives in the general public.

Though Parkinson's is a degenerative condition, taking me out of the classroom as a university professor and away from the sports I love, and has made the activities of daily life very difficult at times, I'm inspired by the people who come into my life and remain in my life who are not afraid to challenge and support me. As my wife says, no matter what challenges I find are in front of me, I should do something scary every once in a while just to test my boundaries. I listened to her, and my life has been full of laughter, a supportive family and, surprisingly, an extended family of good Samaritans. I have found that engagement with the world remains a source of inspiration and always an adventure.

Made in the USA
Monee, IL
17 June 2024

60054482R10128